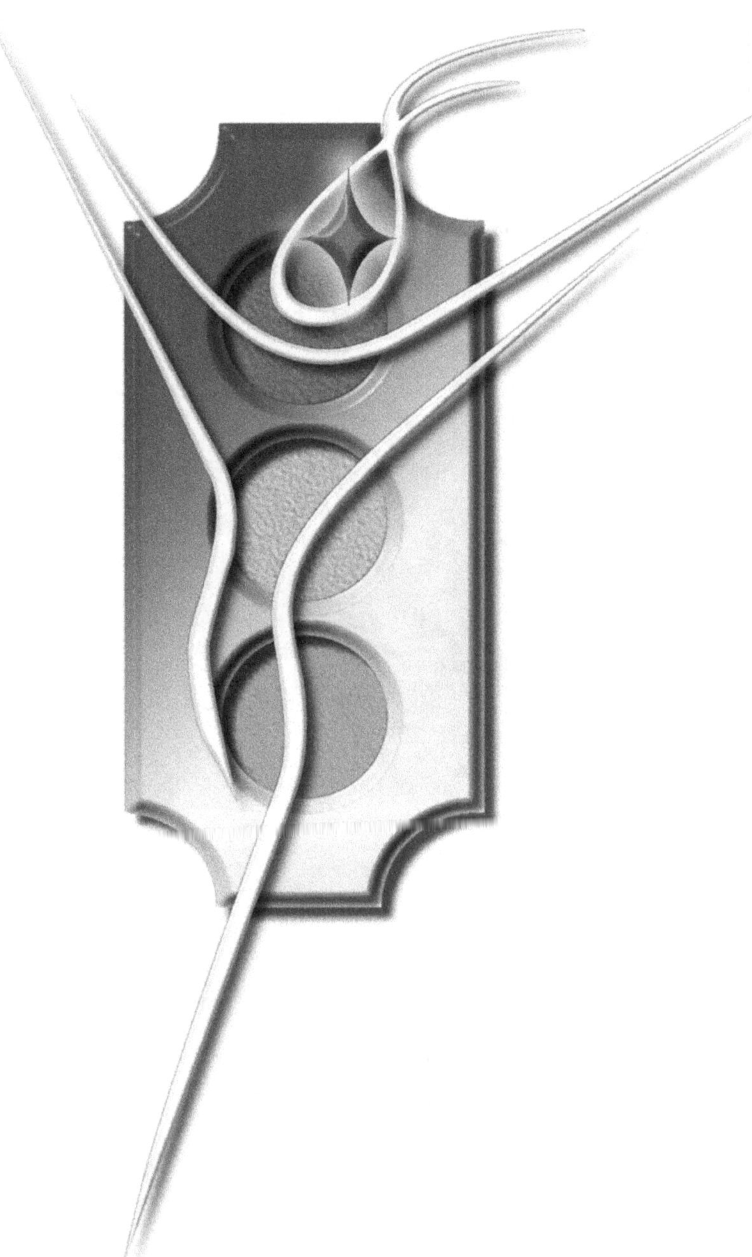

The "Hypothalamus Body Type" is symbolized by a traffic signal. In charge of keeping the body running, they have an intense sense of responsibility, and are therefore cautious about their decisions. They will extensively gather data and focus exclusively on what is at hand.

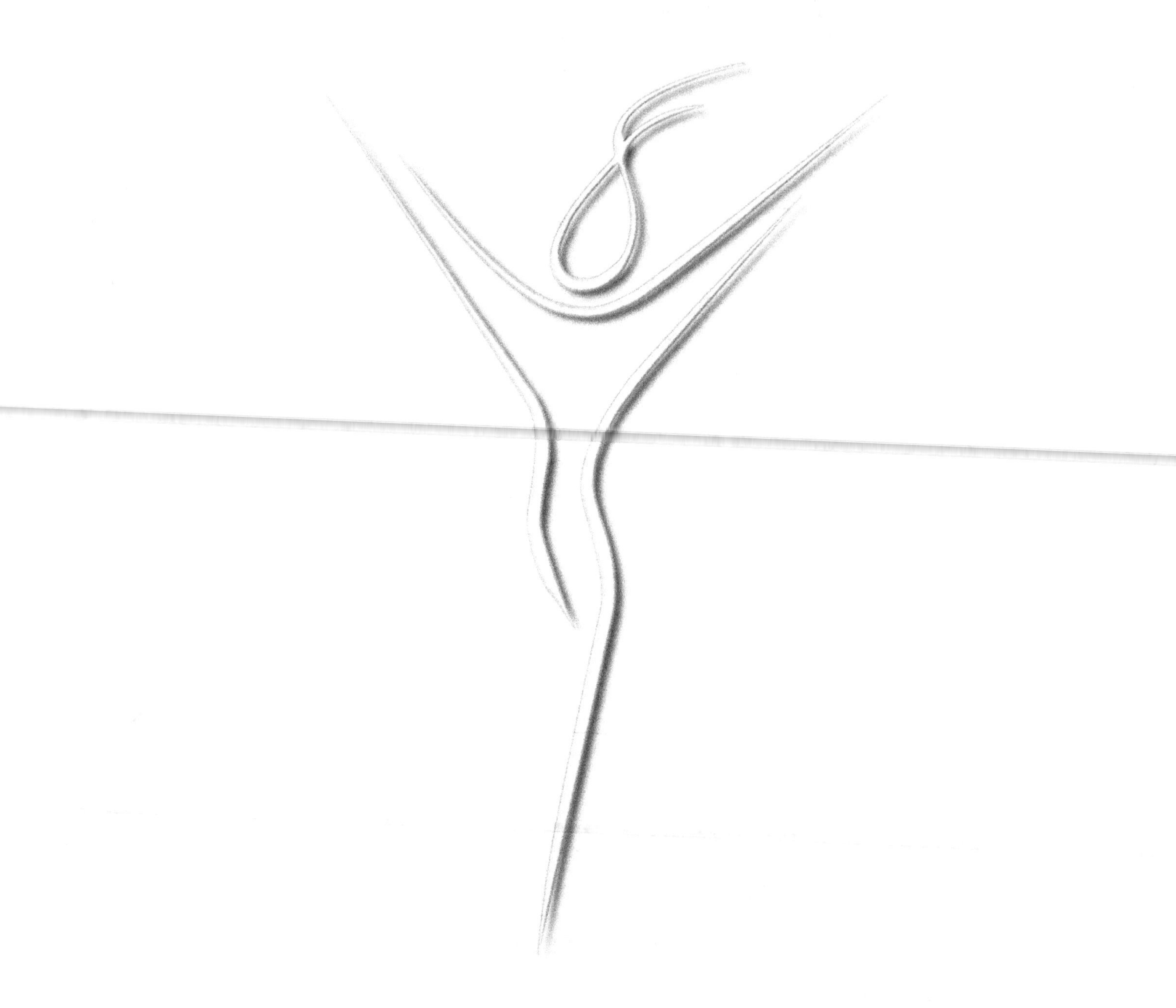

HYPOTHALAMUS PROFILE & DIET

The Ideal Diet — *Does It Exist?*

An *ideal* diet is the one that nutritionally supports *your* specific dietary requirements. It's a way of eating that optimizes your health and vitality as well as normalizing your weight. Most diets are based on the myth that "One Diet Fits All." Many people think that if they can't stay on a diet, it's because they lack willpower. The reality is your body will have food cravings when it doesn't get the nutrients it needs.

The problem with most diets is that they are too general and do not address the specific needs of the individual such as "What time of day do I eat fruit or protein and which vegetables do I eat?" One diet does *not* fit all. Each person has a dominant gland, organ, or system that is stronger than the others which determines weight gain patterns, physical characteristics, and food cravings. This "dominant" gland is the basis of *The 25 Body Type System*™.

Look to *The 25 Body Type System*™ for the diet that truly supports your specific nutritional needs. Following your ideal diet will optimize your health and vitality as well as normalize your weight. Inability to maintain your ideal weight is the first sign of the body being out of balance. *Different Bodies, Different Diets*™ gives you the dietary guidance to optimize your health.

Explanation of Terms and Format

**Location
& Function**

Provides the location and function of the gland, organ, or system associated with each body type. The location is where, when healthy, the majority of the body's energy resides and, when depleted, where the body is most vulnerable.

**Potential Health
Problems**

Identifies the problems your body type is prone to develop when your dominant gland becomes exhausted; includes early warning signs.

**Recommended
Exercise**

Anaerobic exercise is essential for some body types, as it activates the immune system. Surprisingly, this isn't true for all body types. Some types are better with aerobic exercise such as yoga or Tai Chi since this type of exercise serves to rebuild the energy in the body. While exercise has many physical benefits, for most people, its greatest significance is in bringing about emotional well-being. Emotional benefits include releasing stress, clearing or calming the mind, and getting energy moving.

Exercise doesn't have to "look" like exercise. Ordinary daily activities can provide the needed movement required by some types. Included in this exercise section are the types of exercises that provide the greatest benefits.

One of the easiest ways to incorporate exercise is to use a fitness ball as a chair. Sitting on the ball forces you to use your pelvic and lower abdominal muscles. This improves posture and stimulates cerebral-spinal fluid movement, resulting in increased alertness and mental clarity.

**Distinguishing
Features**

These features alone can often be sufficient to differentiate one body type from another. However, not every member of a type necessarily has them, or to the degree where they are strongly evident.

**Additional
Physical
Characteristics**

Supplementary characteristics are useful for comparing and contrasting different body types. Since physical characteristics reflect ethnic and familial heritage as well as dominant and sub-dominant gland characteristics, they can vary considerably. I've described the characteristics that are most commonly seen within each type and noted the ones that tend to run the entire range. For example, height in Liver types can vary from very petite to very tall, even though the majority is of average height. So, *don't rule out a type simply because one or two characteristics don't apply to you.*

**Weight Gain
Areas**

Women: The initial weight gain pattern provides the most important—and often the simplest and most obvious criterion—for determining a woman's body type. Secondary gain refers to any weight gain over 15 pounds.

Men: Describes weight gain as to location and musculature appearance, including areas of primary and secondary weight gain.

Terms and Format

Scheduling Meals

A quick guide for choosing which foods to eat for breakfast, lunch, and dinner, and your ideal meal times.

Choose from the **Healthy** list when you feel strong and healthy, with plenty of energy available to digest your food.

Choose from the **Sensitive** list when your body is under stress (physical, mental or emotional). During these times, energy has been directed elsewhere and is less available for digestion.

Dietary Emphasis

Gives recommendations for weight loss or gain. Lists fat and protein requirements and their best sources. Fats supply essential fatty acids, but not all fats qualify to be included in the minimum fat requirement. Vegetarian diets support some body types, but not all.

Foods High in Amino Acids

Lists the highest sources that are most easily assimilated for your body type. The amino acids threonine, isoleucine and cystine are depleted when a person goes through a lot of changes or personal growth.

Key Supports for System

Suggests foods and/or activities to optimally strengthen or support your particular body type.

Complementary Glandular Support

Identifies the two glands needing to be rebuilt or supported that will give your dominant gland a rest; suggests how this is best accomplished.

Foods Craved

(*When energy is low*) Lists the foods that, by stimulating the body's dominant gland, provide the greatest immediate, but temporary, energy lift.

Foods to Avoid

Identifies foods that are particularly difficult for your body to assimilate, or ones that cause excessive stress.

Recommended Cuisine

The cuisine most supportive to your system—particularly useful when you're dining out and need to select the most appropriate restaurant. Also included are the foods best suited to your type on a daily basis.

Psychological Profile

The Essence embodies the basic nature of each body type. The profile is often the deciding factor in body type identification. Relying on food preferences is often unreliable, since the desire for supporting foods can shift when the dominant gland becomes depleted. Psychological characteristics are often observed from birth and can be useful in identifying a child's body type.

Becoming familiar with the personality parameters of the various body types can help you gain insight into your own personal strengths and challenges, as well as expand your self-awareness. Additionally, aside from better understanding your own basic nature, increasing your knowledge

Terms and Format

Psychological Profile *(cont.)*

about the psychological dimensions of the other body types can enhance your understanding and acceptance of others different from you.

Greater awareness and understanding of yourself provides compassion and understanding of yourself and others. Being aware of the foods you eat and the effect they have on your body is often the first step in self-awareness.

Emotional Issues

While we all have all the emotional patterns, there are some issues that are more of a problem for some types than others. The emotional issues that create the greatest stress are the basic learning challenges for each body type and are listed here along with the other side of the emotion and the affirmation or way of shifting a negative emotional experience to a positive one.

Clearing an emotional pattern is achieved most quickly by connecting and releasing all aspects: the emotional, mental, physical and spiritual.

Feeling both sides of the emotion provides a focus and gives the blocked emotion a positive direction in which to move. Knowing both sides of the emotion allows for a mental understanding and brings the experience into a conscious awareness.

The spiritual aspect is achieved by the transition statement which provides a means of moving from the negative to the positive side of the emotion.

Essential oils access the limbic system of the brain which is the seat of emotion. When essential oils are applied to the alarm points, the cellular memory stored in the body is released.

To clear an emotion, smell the essential oil, feel both sides of the emotion, say the transition statement and apply the appropriate essential oil to the associated alarm point and the emotional release points on the frontal eminences of the forehead. Repeat as needed—whenever the emotion arises or you think about it, as well as at night before going to sleep.

More information is available in ***Releasing Emotional Patterns with Essential Oils,*** also by Carolyn Mein.

Visit ReleasingEmotionalPatterns.com

Physical Profile

Location

At center of brain base, anterior to thalamus and including posterior pituitary.

Function

Controls visceral activities, such as water balance, temperature, and sleep.

Potential Health Problems

Typically, either very healthy or extremely sensitive. Prone to allergies, respiratory, and immune system ailments, high blood pressure, and hearing problems. May be subject to bloating in waist and lower abdomen with fluid retention in upper hips, thighs, and face (especially around eyes). Also vulnerable to digestive distress and sluggish bowels, directly linked to appropriateness of food eaten. Prone to depression and self-destructive thoughts (which can be obsessive).

Recommended Exercise

Exercise is helpful. Its effect is initially physical and can be beneficial in all areas. It facilitates physical integration by providing a way to connect with and feel the physical body. It gives the mind a rest and allows centering to occur. Ideally, exercise 20 minutes every other day, e.g., walking, dancing, singing, callanetics, tennis, basketball, biking, and low impact aerobics. Exercise works best when done recreationally; otherwise, it's low priority.

Women's Characteristics

Distinguishing Features

Height average-to-very tall. Head small-to-average, with long narrow, rectangular, or oval face. Often have wistful, distant look in eyes. Characterized by extremes: will completely immerse themselves in project or endeavor, then transfer all their energy onto something else, going through phases. Generally prefer hot and dry to moderately humid, temperate climate or very cold weather. If prefer hot climate, cold weather drains their energy.

Additional Physical Characteristics

Buttocks relatively flat-to-rounded. Low back curvature straight-to-average. Breasts small-to-average. Shoulders narrower than, to relatively even with, hips. Long, slender torso or broad chest and torso. Waist straight-to-defined. Average to long-waisted. Bone structure medium. Average, elongated musculature. Often have long arms and legs. Feet may be narrow.

Women's Weight Gain Areas

Lower body with initial gain in lower abdomen, entire upper 2/3rds of thighs including upper inner thighs, buttocks, upper hips, and waist. Alternative weight gain pattern: entire abdomen, waist, upper hips, and buttocks. Secondary weight gain in entire abdomen, middle-to entire back, breasts, upper arms, face, and under chin, with little gain in lower hips and legs. May have difficulty gaining or maintaining weight.

Physical Profile

Men's Characteristics

Distinguishing Features

Dominant chest with thick, straight torso and smaller lower body with thin-to-average thighs and calves. Height average to very tall. Characterized by extremes: will completely immerse themselves in a project or endeavor, then transfer all their energy onto something else, as if going through phases. Prefer hot, dry, or moderately humid to temperate climate and dislike cold weather as it drains their energy or prefer the opposite extreme of cold weather.

Additional Physical Characteristics

Buttocks relatively flat-to-rounded. Low back curvature straight-to-average. Shoulders moderately to markedly broader than hips. General appearance is big, usually tall with large torso. Solid musculature in torso with natural protrusion throughout entire abdomen, or entire abdominal paunch. Muscle definition in torso moderate-to-difficult to attain. Bone structure medium-to-large. Hands often large and/or wide, or long and narrow. Feet proportionate, although may be narrow. Long arms and legs. Neck short-to-average. Head small-to-average, with long narrow, rectangular or oval face. May have relatively flat or small occiput (back of head) with limited space from ears to back of head. Hair thin-to-thick. Often have early graying or balding. Hair-loss pattern is frontal with rising forehead, general thinning, or V-shaped with point at center of forehead, marked receding at upper sides and back of head.

Men's Weight Gain Areas

Initial gain in entire abdomen as solid musculature to abdominal paunch, solid thickening in waist, and marked thickening throughout torso. Secondary gain as entire abdominal paunch, thick rolls to solid thickening at waist, increased torso thickening, chest in breast area, face, under chin, and little, if any, gain in hips and thighs. May have difficulty either gaining or losing weight.

Dietary Guidelines

Scheduling "Healthy" Meals

"Healthy" Breakfast: Light, with protein, dairy, and/or fruit.

Healthy Lunch: Moderate, with grain, raw vegetables, legumes, dairy, nuts, and/or seeds

Healthy Dinner: Moderate, with protein, dairy, legumes, cooked or steamed vegetables, and/or grain. Raw vegetables, as in salads, may be eaten with meat and pasta.

"Sensitive" Meals

"Sensitive" Breakfast: Light-to-moderate, with fruit, protein, dairy, and/or grain.

Sensitive Lunch: Moderate, with protein, dairy, and/or vegetables.

Sensitive Dinner: Moderate, with grain, dairy, legumes, and/or vegetables.

Dietary Emphasis

- Raw vegetables best assimilated at lunch; cooked vegetables best for dinner. Broccoli, zucchini or yellow squash should always be eaten raw. Best when more raw than cooked vegetables are consumed. Emphasize cheese, nuts, seeds, and vegetables at lunch. Drink 1/2 gallon of water per day (with or without lemon). In general, good to rotate foods.

- *To detoxify system,* upon arising drink Celestial or herbal tea, or hot water with lemon. Wait 2-3 hours before eating breakfast.

- *For weight loss,* consume 15% of calories from dense protein other than beef or pork, limit fats to 25% of caloric intake with at least 15% from sources listed below under **"Fats"**, limit dairy, frozen yogurt, fried foods, alcohol, caffeine, diet sodas, and breads with yeast, limit snacks to evening, and adhere to food and time schedule. May skip lunch and have light snack at mid-afternoon, or when hungry.

- *For weight gain,* consume protein and fruit for breakfast, increase quantity of food and include snacks, and derive 35% of calories from fats in form of dairy, avocados, nuts, and seeds. Exercise essential to build muscle weight.

- Vegetarian diet recommended when healthy, although diet may consist of up to 20% dense protein.

- Fats, 15-25% for weight loss, 25-30% for maintenance, and 35% for weight gain from avocados, coconuts, seeds (pumpkin, sunflower, and sesame), tahini, and nuts (almonds, pecans, Brazils, macadamias, pistachios, and dry roasted cashews).

Dietary Guidelines

Foods High in Amino Acids

The amino acids threonine, isoleucine and cystine are depleted when a person goes through a lot of changes or personal growth. They are highest and most easily assimilated in turkey, tuna and pumpkin seeds.

Key Support for System

Brown rice, salads, fruits, and vegetables. Eat fruit in morning and, if desired, add mid-morning snack. Kombucha tea and cashews before or after lunch regulate bowels; nuts activate movement. One 8 oz. plain water will often clear headaches or stomachaches. Connect feelings with intellect by nurturing self, through activities such as structured dance or playing musical instrument.

Complementary Glandular Support

Thalamus, through getting sunlight and spending time "communing" with nature; and pituitary, through attempting to understand self, others, or life experiences generally.

Foods Craved

(When Energy is Low) Sweets and fats, such as chocolate, caramel, frozen yogurt, ice cream, chewy cookies, doughnuts, cakes, and pies. *(When feeling heavy or bloated,* may be drawn toward carbonated beverages in attempt to relieve discomfort.)

Foods to Avoid

Ice cream, frozen yogurt, bagels, fried foods, and soft drinks.

Recommended Cuisine

Mexican, Thai, Chinese, Greek, Italian, French. (Prefer simple menus, including grains, noodles, salads, soups, and legumes; unless sensitive, like spicy foods.)

Psychological Profile

Essence

Just as the hypothalamus gland is responsible for and in charge of the involuntary functions necessary for life, including regulating the heartbeat, body temperature, blood pressure, metabolism and blood sugar levels, as well as directing the pituitary gland, Hypothalamus body types have an intense sense of responsibility for their behavior. They seem to be intuitively aware of the significance of their actions, and have a sense of responsibility for accuracy in all they do. Consequently, they approach life with a certain caution. They will generally gather all the necessary tools, study the directions, and formulate a plan before starting a project.

Characteristic Traits

Being single-minded, Hypothalamuses prefer to continue with a task until it is finished or until they reach a saturation point which causes their focus to change. Shifting gears, particularly from mental to emotional, can be difficult, so they prefer not to be interrupted or given multiple tasks.

Characterized by phases, Hypothalamuses will totally immerse themselves in an activity or endeavor, often to the point of becoming a crusader. However, once they complete what they need, they will switch to the next subject that catches their interest. These phases encompass all facets of reality including relationships, new developments, topics, inner probings, travel to unfamiliar places, and career changes.

It's not unusual for men to focus on business, retire, devote themselves to family and home, then abandon retirement to repeat the cycle. They seem most at home in the financial world, often as stock brokers or financial consultants. Money issues are common and they often experience the extremes of abundance and subsistence. Women, however, tend to have a better sense of money management.

With a deep innate curiosity about the nature and function of things, Hypothalamuses are comfortable in the world of concepts and ideas. Their basic strengths include logic, decisiveness, commitment, and determination (essential traits necessary to succeed professionally), especially in the business world. Generally quick thinking and able to see the "big picture" of a project, they tend to work through steps 1-3, then leap ahead to 9-10, delegating to others the intermediate steps.

Motivation

Hypothalamuses travel through different phases as a means of finding themselves. By immersing themselves in their point of interest, they are able to travel to their inner depths and connect integral parts of their being, thereby learning to rely on their own internal guidance rather than conventional standards and opinions. This self-integration is the key to their fulfillment. Although they may not stay focused on an experience or activity for long, while absorbed in something, they experience it fully.

Psychological Profile

The inherent nature of Hypothalamuses is self-contained and independent. Carried to the extreme, it may manifest as difficulties with self-disclosure. This behavior pattern usually forms in childhood with a suppressive family background. Many grew up in homes where their parents were either very critical or overly protective. Sensitive and fearful of failing, making mistakes, or otherwise losing their parents' support or approval, they often felt obliged to inhibit their self-expression. Their natural urges toward exploration of inner and outer worlds thus subdued, they may have developed (at least in the company of others) a certain habit of self-restraint. This is why, if they are to realize their full potential, they must be around people with whom they can feel safe. For the more they're able to experience external support, the more open they'll be about their thoughts and feelings, and the more they'll be able to embrace the changes that can enable them to realize their multifaceted nature.

"At Worst"

At times Hypothalamuses have difficulty trusting their intuition. They may struggle with a problem for too long, trying to solve it logically, without loosening the reins of the intellect to create a space for the solution to manifest. In addition, they may also become stuck in a mental "loop" and fail to move outside themselves. Being mentally focused, they sometimes need other people to serve as sounding boards, particularly if they're to get in touch with what's going on with their own emotions. Focused inward mentally, they are unable to see what others are mirroring back, and remain within the limitations of their own thinking.

Frequently, Hypothalamuses almost seem to expect that outside forces will intervene and take charge of their lives in ways beyond anything they might have imagined. The assumption is that things will magically fall into place without their having to do anything about them. This is frequently the case when it comes to managing money. Hypothalamuses often become so focused on the situation in front of them, such as how to help their children with their immediate desires, that they fail to consider the long term effects of not setting financial boundaries. While they may be very good at managing other people's money, men often fail to do their own financial planning, feeling everything will be okay, so they're free to spend whatever they want. Unfortunately, this is where they can get sidetracked, especially by others. When they listen to outside voices rather than their own inner knowing, they can easily lose their way and fail to experience their abundant zest for life.

Intimate relationships are often a major challenge, women often find they have difficulty maintaining their identity and self-expression, and men have difficulty dealing with problems and sharing their emotions. Unresolved emotional stress usually manifests initially as depression.

Psychological Profile

Alcohol and drugs are commonly used to avoid facing what often seems like problems that have no solution. Work can also be a means of escape, as can finding ways of neglecting an unfulfilling relationship.

"At Best"

Mentally adept, Hypothalamuses are good at analyzing things objectively. Decision-making comes naturally, since they are inclined to understand or relate to things through judging them. Hypothalamuses are effective at handling projects because they can easily grasp what needs to be done, devise an appropriate plan for accomplishing it, and responsibly see the job through. Typically, when embarking on a new project, they'll conscientiously study the written instructions (while other types will bypass them), and learn as much as they can before scrupulously following the plan they have developed.

Having thoroughly investigated a subject before taking action, Hypothalamuses will handle whatever obstacles arise and, if necessary, are comfortable having to redo things later on to achieve their desired results. They are generally receptive and flexible enough to change their approach to something as situations change or if they become aware of a better way of reaching their goals. Hypothalamuses are happiest when they can become creatively absorbed in their current challenge, whether professional or personal.

With active, inquiring minds, they're proficient not only in acquiring but also applying new knowledge. Receptive, sensitive, and intuitive, they are comfortable in the world of concepts and ideas. At times, they will throw themselves into life with intensity, willing to follow their enthusiasm wherever it may lead. While it's their curiosity that drives them to experience the world with immediacy and passion, it's their caution about being physically safe that holds them back. How well they're able to balance these aspects is reflected in the degree of their aliveness. It's when they dance with life that they excel.

At their best, Hypothalamuses are intuitive and receptive. They are able not only to explore and access information, but to manifest it in ways that often take the knowledge to a new level. Once they learn to trust their intuition, they'll rely more on their own internal guidance for answers than on conventional standards or opinions. One of their special gifts is the capacity to get the insights or solutions they require simply by raising a question to themselves and then waiting for the answer to come to them or pop into their head. When they're able to join this innate receptivity or intuitiveness to their inborn tenacity, their success in any endeavor is virtually assured.

Psychological Profile

Emotional Issues

Emotional issues that are basic lessons for the Hypothalamus body type are *shame, fear,* and *betrayal*.

Shame is stored in the hypothalamus which is located between the eyebrows, above the nose. The transitional statement is *"I learn from all of life's experiences."* The other side of shame is **understanding**. Apply the essential oil blend **White Angelica** to the hypothalamus alarm point and frontal eminences.

The opposite of *fear* is **awareness/faith** otherwise described as *"face it"*. The way to access faith/awareness is with the statement *"I face the unknown."* The alarm point for **fear** is the 3rd eye, which is located midline just above the eyebrows half inch above the hypothalamus. The essential oil, **Sandalwood** or **Royal Hawaiian Sandalwood**, is used to hold the frequency of awareness/ faith and is applied to the alarm point and frontal eminences.

Betrayal is ultimately the betrayal of self, although it is most often perceived as betrayal by someone else. The other side of betrayal is **trust**. The transitional statement is *"I have the courage to accept the truth."* The fear of betrayal is stored in the pancreas. The alarm point is located on the left side, below the breast in line with the nipple. The essential oil, **Forgiveness,** is used to release the fear of betrayal; apply to the pancreas alarm point and the emotional points on the frontal eminences.

For a visual location of the alarm points see ***Releasing Emotional Patterns with Essential Oils***, also by Carolyn Mein.

Visit ReleasingEmotionalPatterns.com

Frequency Food Categories

The food lists are divided into 3 categories:

- *Ultra-Support or Frequently Food*s
- *Basic Support or Moderately Foods*
- *Stressful or Rarely Foods*

Frequency of foods refers to the individual food, rather than the entire group. For example, under grains you may eat semolina pasta twice a week, corn once as corn tortillas and once again as corn bread, and rye once as rye crackers and later as rye bread. This way you have your grains and variety.

Ultra-Support or Frequently foods are those that best support your particular body type and can be eaten most often—which means they can be included in three to seven meals per week. When you are hungry and can't think of anything that you especially want to eat, look at your *Frequently* list for ideas. Make sure you get variety from these foods, rather than relying exclusively on the same ones over and over again.

Basic Support or Moderately foods provide variety in your diet. These are the foods you would eat once or twice a week. The lists are designed to be as complete as possible, so don't let unfamiliar foods scare you. You don't have to eat something just because it's listed. However, since no single food contains all the vitamins, minerals, and amino acids, variety is essential. By adding the nutrients from different foods to your diet, you will provide your body with more complete nutrition than you would with a diet of limited food selections.

Stressful or Rarely foods are those that you should eat no more than once a month. While these foods aren't the best for you, the foods you seldom eat aren't usually the ones that cause problems, but rather those that you eat 80 percent of the time. So, being able to eat these *Rarely* foods once in a while eliminates the feeling of deprivation, especially if something you love happens to be on this list.

What happens if you frequently eat *Stressful foods*? They tax your body by taking more energy away than they provide. This is usually done through excessive stimulation of your dominant gland or overloading your digestive system. You will not necessarily experience an immediate stomach ache or headache after eating a stressful food. You could get a delayed reaction, ranging from mild to severe, that could include queasiness, upset stomach, mouth sores, lethargy, fatigue, constipation, diarrhea, dry or burning lips, dry skin, immune system weakness, nervousness, hyperactivity, or a craving for sweets. Symptoms may also be vague or hard to associate with a given food. Weight gain is often the result of eating too many of the *Stressful foods*, since the body will often store what it can't immediately assimilate.

By paying attention to what you are eating, you will eventually get to the point where you will be in tune with what your body needs. Once you are in tune with your body, you will have a good idea of what is best for you to eat or avoid at any given time.

As a small child you had an intuitive sense of what was right for you, as long as you had reasonable choices. At times, such as after a cleansing diet, you probably found it was easier to be aware of which foods you needed and which ones you shouldn't eat. Ideally, we want to recapture our childhood intuition and awareness of our body.

Since the body controls its own metabolic processes, it knows what it needs, and will be your best guide when it comes to what to eat. Your challenge is to correctly interpret the messages your body sends you. Generally, if you don't like a certain food, neither does your body.

Healthy vs. Sensitive Food Lists

Select foods from the *Healthy* food list when you feel strong and healthy. Select foods from the *Sensitive* food list if you have digestive problems, or when you are stressed.

The *Healthy* and *Sensitive* food lists constitute two parameters. Most people fall somewhere between them rather than being completely in one or the other. If you are basically healthy, start with the *Healthy* food list. As you look through it, you will probably find some foods you don't like or don't digest well. If these foods are in the *Ultra Support/Frequently* or *Basic Support/Moderately* category on the *Healthy* list, you will find they have probably been moved to the *Basic Support* or *Stressful* category on the *Sensitive* food list. Use the lists as a guide, being aware that the foods can change categories as your health or awareness changes.

The foods, food combinations, and menus are recommendations—suggestions designed to give you a place to start. Ultimately, you want to be aware of and listen to your body.

Menus: How to Select and Use

Often, menu selections in diet books include foods that don't work for certain people. Their systems might become overloaded by eating too many kinds of foods, or the foods are inappropriate for their body type. This could result in negative symptoms, such as a dull headache, mildly upset stomach, or lack of mental clarity. Another drawback is that the foods these menus recommend often take too much time to prepare. As busy as most of us are, cooking methods should be simple and uncomplicated. Cut down on preparation time by steaming, sautéing, or baking. Instead of rich sauces, season with herbs, combinations of herbs, or small amounts of salt and butter. Focus on menus that are practical. Once you have learned which foods are right for your body type, you can instantly evaluate any recipe as to how it is likely to affect you.

A wide range of menus have been included in this book, so if you run across a food, or food combination you simply cannot eat, cross it off and continue down the list. You are not limited to these menu suggestions, and as you work with the diet, you'll develop your own personal favorites. Quite often there are differences in food choices between types. What one person finds delicious may be downright inedible to another.

Each menu has been tested and approved by numerous members of the same body type. Not only are they tested for taste and desirability, but the food combinations are supportive for this particular type.

Food combinations are an important consideration, because a combination that is good for one type may not be good for another. It's not enough to simply eat protein with any vegetable. Knowing the combinations that are right for you allows you to optimize your diet.

For example, some types can combine almost any vegetable with chicken, while others need to be far more selective. Skin types can add broccoli, cauliflower, carrots, green beans, zucchini, asparagus, chard, mushrooms, or celery, using any one, all or any combinations. Thyroids, on the other hand, can combine broccoli and/or carrots, green beans, or asparagus with chicken, but not all of these at the same time.

You may wonder, is it best to eat your yogurt plain or add fruit? If you are a Pancreas body type, plain is best, but if you are a Pituitary or Kidney, add fruit.

Combinations can be responsible for how well you digest certain foods. Putting together the wrong foods can cause symptoms ranging from mild indigestion, a heavy or sluggish feeling, nausea, bloating, fatigue, irritability, and weight gain to stomachaches and allergic reactions.

Self-testing, or being muscle-tested by another person, can provide a valuable way to determine supportive food combinations. It enables you to determine what your body needs without interference from your conscious mind. Various food combinations can change test results, so when you are figuring out which foods your body really needs, keep asking until you find a combination that tests strong. Please remember that what your body wants today may be different from what it needs tomorrow.

Dietary Categories

Menus are categorized as *Healthy, Weight Loss, Weight Gain,* and *Sensitive.* The menu suggestions for losing weight are often the same as ones recommended for gaining weight, because achieving weight balance requires eating foods that best support your body. You may choose menus from various categories as your dietary requirements change.

Healthy includes all of the menus. It shows your potential, which foods you can eat when you are feeling well, and can be used for general body maintenance. Since it's the ideal diet for your type, it shows you how to get the best nutrition as well as how to combine foods that are especially appropriate for you. Different foods have been combined to complement each other. The criteria are:

1) A strong muscle response when testing them;
2) A positive physical effect after eating them.

Within a particular menu selection you will find food choices in parentheses. This designation means *with or without*—meaning these foods are optional and can be safely deleted from the combination.

Weight Loss menus are designed to be low fat and low calorie, paying particular attention to specific body type requirements. They often revolve around foods that help to detoxify the body, and include protein that is easily assimilated for rebuilding.

Weight Gain is for that neglected portion of the population rarely acknowledged as having a problem, specifically those who have difficulty maintaining adequate weight. People in this group are generally sensitive or have health problems interfering with assimilation. Also included here are athletes wanting to build muscle mass and people recovering from illness.

Sensitive menus are planned around the ***Sensitive*** food list. These foods provide the greatest support and are the most easily digested. Originally developed for people who had severely depleted their bodies or were extremely sensitive, these menus are to be used when you don't feel well, are recovering from an illness, or are under a lot of stress. If you find yourself in the ***Sensitive*** category, realize that as your system gets stronger, your foods will expand into the ***Healthy*** list.

Your body becomes extremely sensitive when it has been severely stressed—usually from chronic illness, prolonged fatigue, sleep deprivation, poor digestion or assimilation, hypoglycemia or low blood sugar, or as a result of obesity. This is when the sensitive diet is warranted. The basic sensitive diet, common to all the types, consists mostly of protein and vegetables. At times it will involve cutting down or eliminating sugars, including fruits, carbohydrates, and possibly reducing the grains down to only basmati rice.

One way to assist your carbohydrate metabolism is to give your pancreas a rest by restricting your carbohydrate and sugar consumption to a period of less than one hour a day. This allows the pancreas to secrete insulin only once, thus reducing stress on the body. Body types prone to pancreas exhaustion are the Pancreas and Skin types.

Some menus include ***Very Sensitive***, for people with extremely sensitive digestive systems.

The diets provided for the various body types are meant as a guide and can be modified to best suit your needs and desires. While your body is constantly adapting to changing conditions, the kind and quantity of food you choose to eat will vary with your activities.

Foods required to support your body during physical activity will differ from what is needed to support your brain during mental activity. Also, the amount of food you need at a particular time depends on what you are doing. If you are vigorously exercising, you will need to eat more than if you are sitting at a desk. The quantity of food eaten at meals will vary, as well as the choice of foods.

Example: Thyroid types can eat from almost any of the food groups during the day and in varying amounts, depending on how active they are. Those who expend a lot of mental energy during the day do best with a moderate breakfast of protein with a vegetable or grain, possibly followed by fruit juice or tea.

A mid-afternoon snack is desirable if you eat dinner late. The size and time of the evening meal often determines whether a heavy breakfast is wanted the next morning.

Regardless of your body type, it is important to change your diet appropriately when you are trying to heal, or when you are under stress. You should also adjust it if you increase your activity level, or if you change your environment.

Cleanse

A cleanse day is included with the one week sample menus to give your body a rest and chance to flush toxins. Cleanse duration can vary from one to three days, and you can change the frequency from weekly to every other week, or monthly, depending on your body and state of health. The menu itself will often include a variety of ways to prepare the food: steamed, raw and/or juiced. You can try any of the choices or vary them from week to week.

Ideally, on a Cleanse Day you give your body time to rest and pamper yourself. Just do what you feel like doing. It is helpful initially to visualize what you would like your life to be like five years from now—what you'll be like if you continue on the path you are on, and then see yourself making the changes you need to have the life you would like. This is also a good time to work on emotional issues associated with your body type.

Emotional Clearing

Each body type has certain core issues that are predominant. Even though we all have all the emotions, each body type has different lessons or challenges to work through. The core issue for your particular body type is listed at the end of the psychological profile. Another way to identify an emotional pattern is to read the "At Worst" section of the psychological profile. If you relate to a trait(s), refer to *Releasing Emotional Patterns with Essential Oils* for step-by-step instructions on clearing and releasing your core issues.

Relaxation Exercise

For a one minute relaxation that can be done as frequently as desired, close your eyes, relax your eyes and tongue. Focus your attention on your heart, see and feel a golden light coming from your heart and radiating out to all parts of your body.

If I follow the diet, what can I expect?

Stand before a full-length mirror in your underwear or a bathing suit. Turn and observe yourself from all angles: front, back, and side views. Take a careful look. Where do you appear to have excess weight? Do some areas look out of proportion, while others seem just right? Or maybe you need to put on a little weight in certain parts of your body?

The weight you carry on your body is a good reflection of how your system uses the food you eat. Eating the foods that are right for your particular body type and also observing the times of the day when these will be most effective for your system will enable you to give your body just what it needs.

This "conscious" eating will cause your body to lose unnecessary weight so that your system can function properly without the mental and physical stress of dieting. And, if you want to gain weight, it will be much easier as you will know what to eat as well as the times of the day when your system will get the best results from your food intake.

Eating for your body type is different from the usual weight loss diets, because now you are supplying your system with foods that truly support it. Weight loss diets usually stress deprivation of some kind, which often causes a rebound effect when you go off the diet. Eating the right foods for your body type allows you to reach and then maintain your correct body weight. This, in itself, is a step towards optimal health.

The most common comment I hear from patients who have begun to follow the diet for their body type, is "I feel better!" Many tell me that they have a higher energy level and that they no longer feel hungry between meals. Some are better able to avoid the sweets and caffeine that they were dependent on for that little boost they needed to get them through the day. Often they are able to accomplish much more because of better endurance, and they have more energy at the end of the day.

What it really comes down to is this: If you follow the eating regimen tailored to your particular body type, you will be using food the way nature, or your special nature, meant you to. When you support your body with a diet plan best suited for it, you can achieve an optimal state of physical health and well-being.

You must eat in order to live, so why not eat those foods that enliven you, unlocking the stores of energy and vitality that you may never have known before. And, with it, you can maintain that energy flow as it constantly replenishes and rebuilds your system.

Weight Loss Tips

Since gaining weight is often the first symptom of an imbalance in the body, the initial step to losing weight is to rebalance your body. The *Healthy* and *Sensitive* diets are designed to accomplish this goal. Occasionally, when people begin eating the foods they have deprived themselves of (sometimes for years), they put on weight. It's not uncommon to experience an increase in appetite for a short period before the system stabilizes.

There are a couple of pitfalls I'd like to caution you about. Some types have a strong tendency to *go overboard on certain foods*, especially if they have been depriving themselves of them. If the foods happen to be high fat or high calorie, weight gain can result, particularly if the diet is not adjusted accordingly.

The next common problem is *quantity of food*. The amount you eat is left to your discretion, as it will vary according to your activities and diet earlier in the day or week. Naturally, if you have been eating large meals, you may be ready for less food. However, if your food consumption has been low, your body may be needing more fuel.

Another cause of weight gain relates to *muscle rebuilding*. When the body is robbed of adequate nutrients, it may consume muscle and replace it with fat. Later, this lost muscle must be replaced and fat eliminated. Dieters sometimes notice they weigh more after decreasing their fat intake and increasing their activity level. This is because all that rebuilt muscle weighs more than fat—so, it's best not to rely solely on the scale. Remember, fat takes up more room than muscle, so when you've lost fat, your clothes feel loose, even though your body weight may increase.

Generally speaking, two weeks on the *Healthy* diet is sufficient to provide the nutrients that may have been missing and to adequately support complementary systems, enabling the body to rebuild. Then the actual dieting can begin, employing the weight loss menus.

Emotional Eating

Are you overeating because you feel hollow inside? Do you use food, especially sweets, to reward yourself? Are these foods—particularly salty or fatty snacks—a necessary part of any social event? Do you nurture yourself with food? Do you use excess weight as a buffer? If you answered yes, and frequently, to any of these questions, you may want to check for an underlying emotional component. Negative emotions are fairly easy to recognize; fearing the negative consequences of expressing them, you might have a tendency to stuff these feelings, only to have them eventually surface. Since neither stuffing nor expressing negative feelings are viable options, you need a way to express them positively. The goal is to identify the positive emotion, access it, and express it.

All too often, even when we know the positive side of an emotion, we are so caught up in our negative programming we are unable to access it. Let's take anger for example: the positive side of anger is laughter. While laughter is a positive emotion, it can be surrounded by negative experiences. Therefore, being able to access the positive side of the emotion of anger as well as laughter requires clearing the negative energy around both.

Clearing an emotional pattern requires being able to access both sides of the emotion, understand the situation where it was created, learn its lesson, and then clear it out of cellular memory. Additional instructions for this process can be found in *Releasing Emotional Patterns with Essential Oils,* also by Carolyn Mein.

Conquering Food Cravings

Why is it that you sometimes have this awful, insatiable desire for a certain food at a particular time? Lemon meringue pie after a big meal, or a soft drink in the middle of the afternoon, or dill pickles when you are pregnant? What causes a craving, and how should you deal with it?

Food cravings usually involve your dominant gland and its need for stimulation. In order to overcome the craving, you need to understand what your body really wants. The urge to eat certain foods could be caused by emotional stress, or the need for specific nutrients missing from your diet. For example, the Thyroid body type craves sweets and carbohydrates because these are the foods that best stimulate the thyroid gland. When the body is stressed, the dominant gland—in this case, the thyroid—comes to the rescue and will continue to do so until exhausted and unable to respond. Once exhausted, symptoms of thyroid problems appear. In the meantime, the body craves foods that it knows will provide the greatest stimulation and the quickest energy lift.

Giving in to your food cravings will eventually cause you to overload your dominant gland, and put undue stress on your system. The way out of this dilemma is to understand why you crave a certain food and what your body is really saying with the craving. Basic nutritional needs are the basis for food cravings, so when you can determine what your system really needs, you can respond to this need in a way that supports your dominant gland as well as your body. Once you begin choosing the right foods in place of those that only stimulate, you are well on your way to achieving a healthy balance in your system.

Sugar Cravings

Craving sugar? (Sugar includes not only chocolate, candy or sweets, but also sweet fruit and carbohydrates like breads or muffins.) A desire for sugar is one of the first indications of protein deficiency. It's also common to crave sweets after eating too much protein. Since sugar is needed to get protein across the blood-brain barrier, a sugar craving could be your body's signal that you need to assimilate more protein.

Eating sugar, in any form, stimulates the thyroid gland, which controls metabolism. While you might feel more energetic immediately after eating sugar, its consumption leads to problems in the long run, because the underlying situation has not been properly addressed.

An energy drop, which often initiates sugar cravings, comes from adrenal insufficiency—often the result of fatigue or exhaustion. Rebuilding the adrenals requires protein and vitamin C. The protein most readily utilized is dense protein from sources like fish, chicken, turkey, and eggs, as opposed to vegetable protein like beans and other legumes. Broth-based soups are another easy way to assimilate dense protein.

Some people think they will benefit by increasing the amount of sweet fruits in their diet, citing their high vitamin C content. However, sweet fruit contains a lot of thyroid-stimulating fructose, which taxes the adrenals. Vegetables such as red bell peppers and broccoli can be better vitamin C alternatives. Focus on protein and vegetables for rebuilding the adrenals.

Artificial Sweeteners

You have been told you need to reduce your sugar and that refined sugar is bad because it robs the body of nutrients—so you think artificial sweeteners might be a good choice, right? *Wrong.*

The wood alcohol in the artificial sweetener, aspartame, converts to formaldehyde and then to formic acid, which in turn causes metabolic acidosis when its temperature exceeds 86 degrees Fahrenheit. Aspartame is marketed as Nutra Sweet®, Equal® and Spoonful®. In her lecture on aspartame, presented to the World Environmental Conference in 1997, Nancy Markle reported that methanol toxicity mimics multiple sclerosis, triggering systemic lupus and fibromyalgia symptoms. Some of the best sources of methanol toxicity are Diet Coke® and Diet Pepsi®.

Aspartame is not a diet product! The Congressional record said that it could make you crave carbohydrates and make you FAT. Dr. Roberts stated that when he got patients off aspartame, their average weight loss was 19 pounds per person. Formaldehyde stores in the fat cells, particularly in the hips and thighs. For web site addresses and more information on aspartame, check the *Resources*.

Food Assimilation and Weight Management

In order for a food to be considered a food, it has to contain fat, protein, and carbohydrates—even if the quantity is too small to appear on package labels. If any of these components are missing, the body doesn't register the substance as a food and won't assimilate it. Foods are classified based on their dominant component: fat, protein, or carbohydrate; e.g., meat is a protein, butter is a fat, and fruits, vegetables and grains are carbohydrates.

The assimilation of these foods, however, still depends upon the presence of all three components—fat, protein, and carbohydrates. Without them, digestion and assimilation are incomplete, which, of course, leads to a system imbalance.

Anything consumed that your body can't identify as being a food is considered toxic and treated accordingly. Too much of a toxic substance will overload the liver and may trigger a migraine headache or cause headaches in general. Sometimes the body will keep the toxic substance in fluid suspension, resulting in bloating or fluid retention. It may also be stored in fat cells.

Carbohydrates, which break down into sugar, are necessary for protein assimilation. This became quite evident when I began testing a product called Re-Vita®.

Re-Vita®

Re-Vita is a complete protein and contains all 22 amino acids. Initially, reading the ingredients, I was rather skeptical of its value, since the first ingredient listed was fructose (a sugar), and the main component was spirulina, an algae that few people are able to assimilate. Another ingredient was ginseng—an herb mostly considered beneficial for men, but not necessarily for women.

I was pleasantly surprised when I discovered that 70-80% of my patients, most of whom were very sensitive nutritionally, responded well to Re-Vita. I later learned that sugar was an essential factor in making this product easy to assimilate. Sugar enables protein to pass through a membrane between the bloodstream and the brain cells known as the blood/brain barrier. It also allows the same process to occur in other cells. So, Re-Vita duplicates what is naturally found in nature by using the fructose (sugar) to assimilate the protein (amino acids). This is also true for other sources of protein. It explains why carbohydrates are found in combination with protein in whole foods, and why we desire something sweet after a high protein meal.

Proper assimilation of food also requires the presence of vitamins and minerals, which are often deficient in processed foods. A vitamin and mineral supplement sometimes helps to provide these essentials, but knowing which supplements to use requires an understanding of the body's needs. Muscle testing is helpful in making the right selection.

Most vitamin companies manufacture a multiple vitamin/mineral supplement, but in more than twenty years of testing, I hadn't found one that was right for most people until I found Re-Vita. In addition to amino acids, Re-Vita contains vitamins, minerals, as well as trace minerals in a form that is easy to assimilate.

Most minerals are simply mined from the earth and put into capsules. Unfortunately, our bodies aren't designed to assimilate them in this form. Plants can convert minerals straight from the ground, but we can't. We can absorb them after the plants have converted them, or from animals who have digested the plants. If the plants don't absorb the minerals, they can't pass them on to us. This is why the algae used in Re-Vita is fed minerals, and why we assimilate minerals best from food sources.

Re-Vita is different in that the assimilation is made possible by feeding the minerals to spirulina rather than simply adding them to the formula. The algae then process the minerals into a form easily absorbed by the human body.

Food activates the digestive process. If vitamin pills are swallowed on an empty stomach, the stomach has no way of interpreting what's there. This is why the majority of nutritional supplements are most effective when taken with food. Consequently, mixing Re-Vita with food maximizes its effectiveness.

Popular Ways to Use Re-Vita®

*Use Revita in **Grains** as a:*

- sweetener on cereal like oatmeal, cream of rye or rice
- syrup on pancakes, waffles, or French toast
- flavoring for popcorn or in trail mix
- cookie—by melting butter, mixing oat flour, salt to taste, and Re-Vita, then adding fine cut raw oatmeal. Proportions vary depending on quantity and the consistency you prefer for your cookie. *(To make it stick together, forming a flat patty or ball, requires more butter. If you'd rather have it crumbly and eat it with a spoon, or use it as a topping over fruit or yogurt, use less butter.)*

*Use Revita in **Fruit** as a:*

- juice sweetener—add with water to unsweetened cranberry concentrate
- sweetener over cherries, rhubarb, or any other tart fruit. *(May also be used as the sweetener in fruit desserts)*
- lemonade—one lemon or two or three limes and one packet of Lemon/Lime Revita to one quart water (may drink exclusively for one to three days as a cleanse)

*Use Revita in **Dairy** as a:*

- sweetener and flavor for your favorite dairy product, such as yogurt, kefir, or milk (may add nuts, ie. pecans, pine nuts or almonds)
- coffee—adding 1/8 teaspoon of chocolate flavor to a cup of coffee will replace the nutrients depleted by the coffee

*On **Vegetables:***

- use Revita over squash or pumpkin

Basically, use Re-Vita as a sweetener on anything else that appeals to you. To obtain Re-Vita, see *Resources*.

Fats and Cholesterol

The body manufactures 70-90% of the cholesterol found in your blood stream. It uses cholesterol to manufacture hormones, antibodies and enzymes. Since enzymes are killed at 110°, cooked foods are enzyme deficient. To digest cooked food the body must then supply the needed enzymes. If the body is unable to digest what was eaten, it sends a signal to the liver to manufacture more cholesterol which is used to manufacture more enzymes. However, since the poorly digested food creates more stress on the body, the body often manufactures more hormones which it then stores as fat.

Hormones are manufactured in response to stress. Since the additional hormones are not exactly what the body needs, it stores them in the same regions it did during adolescence, i.e., as fat— leading to weight gain in specific regions, determined by your body type.

There is a lot of confusion around fats. Since fats contain more calories than protein and carbohydrates, many diets focus on the reduction of fats to reduce calories. Simply cutting out all fats or eating just any fat won't help, because you're not getting the essential fatty acids you need. This in turn triggers your body to produce more cholesterol, which leads to weight gain. Hormonal imbalances, such as hot flashes and mood swings, are often the result of a lack of essential fatty acids. Ideal sources for essential fatty acids your body can best utilize can be found under *Dietary Guidelines*.

Margarine vs. Butter

Butter is an excellent source of essential fatty acids, while margarine has been proven to have negative affects. Margarine is a product of hydrogenation, which produces trans fats—molecules that are harmful to the body's cell structure. These *trans fatty acid compounds* (TFA's) raise the levels of harmful cholesterol (LDL) and have been directly linked to increased risk of coronary disease, cancer and stroke.

Margarine is not the only source of trans fats. They are often found in breads, muffins, rolls, flour tortillas, breakfast cereals, cookies, peanut butter, chips and crackers. Trans fats are found in any product containing hydrogenated or partially hydrogenated oils. These products are often advertised as containing no cholesterol and include fake eggs, shortening, coffee creamers, and fried foods.

Heating liquid vegetable oils in the presence of metal catalysts and hydrogen produces trans fats. Processed food manufacturers and fast food makers prefer hydrogenated oils over unsaturated vegetable oils because they are solid at room temperature, have a longer shelf life and allow for high-temperature frying.

A comprehensive review of scientific evidence published in the June 24, 1999, issue of the *New England Journal of Medicine* confirms the connection between trans fats and coronary heart disease through their deleterious effects on cholesterol. Though trans fats do not contain cholesterol, they have an unhealthy effect on this substance once inside the body, raising the LDL, or "bad" cholesterol and lowering the "good" HDL cholesterol. This effect is essentially a double whammy for your arteries. Because these fats increase the bad while lowering the good cholesterol, it is estimated that the negative effect of eating them is about double that of saturated fats.

FAT: Total % of Fat Grams and Calories per Day

Total Calories per day	20%		25%		30%		35%		40%	
	Grams	Calories	Grams	Calories	grams	calories	grams	calories	grams	calories
1000	22	200	27	250	33	300	38	350	44	400
1500	33	300	41	375	50	450	58	525	66	600
1800	40	360	50	450	60	540	70	630	80	720
2000	44	400	56	500	67	600	77	700	88	800
2200	49	440	60	550	73	660	85	770	98	880

PROTEIN: Total % of Protein Grams and Calories per Day

Total Calories per day	20%		25%		30%		35%		40%	
	grams	calories	grams	calories	grams	calories	grams	calories	grams	calories
1000	50	200	62	250	75	300	87	350	100	400
1500	75	300	93	375	112	450	131	525	150	600
1800	90	360	112	450	135	540	157	630	180	720
2000	100	400	125	500	150	600	175	700	200	800
2200	110	440	137	550	165	660	192	770	220	880

How Much Fat and Protein?

Many diets emphasize low fat or low protein; as a result, I see many people who are fat and protein deficient. The average requirements I see are 25-30% fat and approximately 30% protein.

We have been told we need to reduce our food intake to 1000 to 1500 calories for weight loss. With weight being a chronic issue, I see many women who need to rebuild their bodies and initially require 1800 calories. Men generally require 2000 calories—and more if they do a lot of physical labor or exercise.

The table at the top of the page shows the number of calories and grams of fat based on percentage of calories from fats and the total number of calories consumed. The next table shows the same information for protein. On the following page are typical food examples with their gram and calorie content.

There are, however, some types, such as the Stomach body type, who need to reduce their fats to 20% to lose weight. Conversely, types like Gallbladder and Eye gain weight if their fat intake falls below 20-25%. Weight loss requirements can be quite specific, since not all fat sources are the same, and each body type has its specific sources from which to derive fat. This specific information is included in the *Dietary Guidelines Summary* section under *Fats*.

Fat, Protein and Calorie Content of Common Foods

FATS	Fat Grams	Protein Grams	Cal.
1 oz. almonds, dry roasted	14.7	4.6	167
1 med. avocado	30.8	4	324
1 oz. Brazil nuts	18.8	4.1	186
1 oz. Brie cheese	7.9	5.9	95
1 tsp. butter	3.8	<0.1	34
1 oz. cashews, dry roasted	13.2	4.4	163
1 oz. Cheddar cheese	9.4	7.1	114
1 oz. coconut, dry & unsweetened	18.3	2	187
1 oz. cottage cheese	1.3	3.5	29
1 oz. cream cheese	9.9	2.1	99
1 oz. feta cheese	6	4	75
1 oz. kefir, plain	1	1	19
1 oz. mozzarella, part skim milk	4.5	6.9	7
1 tbs. olive oil	14	0	120
1 tbs. peanut butter	7	4	90
1 oz. pumpkin seeds, roasted	12	9.4	148
1 oz. ricotta, part skim milk	2.2	3.2	39
1 oz. sesame seeds	14.1	5	162
1 oz. sunflower seeds	14.1	6.5	162
1 oz. Swiss cheese	7	8	100
1 oz. tahini sesame butter	14.5	5.1	169
8 oz. yogurt, plain, low fat	3.5	11.9	144

PROTEIN	Fat Grams	Protein Grams	Cal.
6 oz. fresh rainbow trout	7	45	257
6 oz. halibut	5	45	239
6 oz. haddock	2	41	190
6 oz. flat fish sole, flounder	3	41	200
6 oz. salmon	13	47	315
6 oz. shrimp	2	36	168
6 oz. light tuna packed in water	1	51	222
6 oz. roasted chicken dark meat, no skin	17	47	348
6 oz. roasted chicken breast meat, no skin	6	53	281
6 oz. roasted turkey dark meat, no skin	12	49	318
6 oz. roasted turkey white meat, no skin	6	51	277
6 oz. lamb chops lean, broiled	17	51	368
6 oz. center pork chops lean, broiled	18	54	393
6 oz. leg of lamb	13	48	326
6 oz. T-bone steak	36	42	507
6 oz. Porterhous steak	36	42	519
6 oz. roasted tenderloin	47	40	600
6 oz. round tip	30	44	467
6 oz. top sirloin	29	47	458
2 oz. 1 beef frankfurter	17	7	184
1 egg, large	5	6.3	75

Source: *The Corinne Netzer Encyclopedia of Food Values,* Corinne T. Netzer, N.Y.: Dell Books, 1992

Even though your diet may call for 25-35% of your total calories from protein, the amount of protein per day may vary. For example, you may be really hungry one day and eat more protein, maybe even 50%, then feel like eating only vegetables the next day. The recommended percentage is designed to give you a realistic guideline to be used as a dietary average. This gives you flexibility and allows you the freedom to ultimately learn to listen to your body.

To make sure you are getting the essential fatty acids you need, choose the majority of your fats from your best sources listed under *Fats* in the *Dietary Guidelines* section.

Snacks

For most body types, nuts and seeds are included among the best fat sources. Because they contain primarily fat and protein, nuts and seeds are excellent snacks. They provide quick energy and are easy to carry with you.

Roasted, unsalted nuts and seeds are usually easiest to digest and can be kept for extended periods of time in your car, purse, briefcase or desk. Unfortunately, the roasting process does kill enzymes. While eating them raw would be the best, most people have difficulty assimilating very many raw nuts and seeds unless they are soaked. Soaking activates the enzymes and helps remove acids, making them much easier to digest.

To soak, simply put some almonds, pumpkin or sunflower seeds in a bowl and cover with your drinking water. Let stand for 12 to 24 hours, then pour off the water (you can use it to water your plants). Take the quantity you want for the day and save the rest for later. Soaked nuts and seeds can begin to mold if stored at room temperature in a plastic bag for too long. However, they will keep for several days in your refrigerator.

Fruits

Dried fruit is easy to keep in your desk or carry in your purse. Taking fresh fruit and vegetables requires a little more forethought, but it's well worth the effort. Keeping your blood sugar levels up will keep you from grabbing a candy bar or overeating at the next meal.

Vegetables

Having trouble eating your vegetables, or getting your children to eat them? How old are they? If you are buying them from the supermarket, chances are it has been more than a week since they were picked. The life force in plants is highest when they are ready to be picked, not before. Once picked, they start to lose their life force or vital energy, so you want to eat above-ground vegetables within a week from the time they are picked, and ideally as soon after picking as possible. Root vegetables like potatoes hold energy longer. The greatest value of fresh food is its life force energy.

How fresh is your produce? When was it picked and how long has it been on the shelf or in your refrigerator? If your vegetables don't taste good to you and you are having difficulty eating them, check to see how fresh they really are.

Another cause of vitality loss in food is overcooking. What do you do if you can't get really fresh produce? Frozen vegetables often are the best alternative.

Amino Acids

The amino acids threonine, isoleucine and cystine are depleted when a person goes through a lot of changes or personal growth. The best sources are found in the ***Dietary Guidelines*** section.

Water

Our bodies are made up primarily of water. Consequently, the right kind of water in adequate quantities is essential. Approximately one-half gallon of water per day is ideal for most people. This sounds like a lot but it is only eight 8-ounce or four 16-ounce glasses. The Kidney body type often requires a little less, but most types need between 1-1/2 quarts and 3/4 gallon of water daily. If you live in a hot, dry climate or are especially active during the day, your requirements may increase.

Drinking water will curb your appetite. Many people eat, not because they are really hungry, but because they are dehydrated. In addition to flushing the toxins out of the body, water can help burn calories by metabolizing stored fat. Many people think that because a beverage contains water, it counts as water. Unfortunately, this is not true. The body registers liquids like coffee, fruit juice, soft drinks, soups, etc. as food. So, if you are drinking anything other than plain water, even though it contains water, the body can't use it as water.

The kind of water you drink will determine how easy it is for you to drink enough water. Heavily chlorinated water from the tap not only doesn't taste good but also adds toxic substances to your body. Since the main reason to drink water is to cleanse your system, drinking anything other than pure water is counter-productive. The best waters contain some minerals. This is why drinking water from a fresh mountain stream can taste so good. Distilled water leaches minerals, as can water filtered through reverse osmosis.

One way to upgrade water is to add a small amount of juice such as lemon, lime, apple, or grape. Sometimes this is enough to balance its mineral content and improve the taste. When you are dining in restaurants or traveling and must drink water from an unknown source, adding the juice of a lemon slice will help improve the taste and neutralize the chlorine, as well as other toxic substances. Adding a drop or two of peppermint oil will also upgrade water and aid digestion. Drinking peppermint water during air travel not only improves the taste of the water, but because it has anti-bacterial, anti-fungal and anti-viral properties, breathing the peppermint as you are drinking it can help protect you from air-borne microbes.

The best indication of whether a water is good for you is taste. If you don't like the taste of a particular water, it usually isn't the one that's right for you. It's easy to drink water when you like the taste. Muscle testing can also be used to determine your best water source.

Dietary Changes: "Take it Slow"

Listening to your body is being sensitive to your body's reactions to the foods you eat. This is important in making changes in your diet and also in starting special diets. Sudden changes in what you eat, even when you go from a poor diet to a healthful one, can produce negative effects in your system.

For example, when a person's system has deteriorated, whole, unrefined foods are usually indigestible. The body simply cannot tolerate a sudden change to a more healthful diet. A system that is used to highly refined junk food needs the fats and sugars that are easily metabolized for quick energy. These are stimulants that keep the system going but, at the same time, destroy health. If an individual is eating junk food, especially a child or a teenager, changing their diet should be done gradually. The body must be given time to adjust to new foods and eating patterns and to rebuild the weakened systems.

When foods can't be assimilated by an unbalanced system, switching to a healthful diet can leave the person devoid of energy. This alone could encourage one to abandon the diet and go back to unhealthy eating, which at least will supply the energy necessary to function.

So, before making any serious dietary changes, it is important to carefully consider what you are presently eating. Major changes usually need to be made in small steps, and care should be taken to eat those foods that will restore the depleted system.

Maintaining Your Diet

These diets are neither fads nor instant cures. It's about making permanent, long-term change. This lifetime eating program is based on sound dietary practices and what is individually right for each body type.

To get the greatest value out of your specific eating program, you'll need to change your eating patterns to the ways that truly support your body. In this process you will become more aware of when changes are necessary. Once you experience what it's like to feel really healthy, you will also know when your body is out of balance as well as how to regain that balance.

Long-term change rarely happens overnight, yet changing your eating habits can bring you better health and a more fulfilling lifestyle. Here's how some of my patients began to incorporate this program into their lifestyles:

> *"I looked at the diet, familiarized myself with what was ideal for me, and then compared it to what I was currently doing. I incorporated the parts that were easy for me, adding a single item I was attracted to, and put the diet away until I was ready for more."*

> *"I worked on one part at a time, first the foods, then the meals. The foods meant adding or deleting certain foods. Meals involved using new menus, mainly at breakfast."*

"I changed a pattern of eating sweets, like ice cream, cookies, candy, or pastries, from anytime during the day to only when my body could easily handle them. Now I save the sweets for later and if I still want them, eat them as an evening or bedtime snack."

"I shifted the time of day that I ate my largest meal from dinner to lunch time. It dramatically changed my energy level." (Pineal, Medulla, Skin, Pancreas, and Gallbladder types will definitely relate to this.)

"I followed the diet for 2 or 3 weeks and noted how I felt. Then I went back to the old way and noted the difference. I am convinced that it is definitely worth the effort to establish new patterns".

"I added balancing foods. As a Medulla type, I found I could comfortably eat pepperoni pizza if I drank pineapple/coconut juice after it."

"I started keeping a diary of what I ate and how I felt after each meal. I read my diary while I'm riding my stationary bicycle. This motivates me to stay with my diet and keeps me from sliding back into my old habits. When I first started following my diet a year ago, I felt great. Then I felt I was invincible and could eat anything. It worked for a while, but then I gradually started slipping back into my old habits. My headaches returned, my energy was down, and I became irritable and short-tempered. I went back on my diet and felt dramatically better. That's when I realized I needed to keep a diary to keep reminding me that I can feel great and what it takes to do it."

"Not everyone in my family is the same type..."

Rarely is every member of the family the same body type. Couples are often complementary types, sometimes opposites, and on occasion (usually with Pineals, Pituitaries, Stomachs, and Adrenals) the same. Perhaps one, and sometimes more than one child will be the same type as one of the parents. Most often body types in a family will be similar, and generally compatible—meaning that types corresponding to glands found in the head, such as the Pineal, are often attracted to similar types, such as the Thyroid, or to types whose dominant systems encompass the entire body, such as the Lymph, Blood, or Nervous System. To give additional examples, the Thalamus is quite compatible with the Hypothalamus, as is the Liver with the Kidney, Gallbladder, and Pancreas. Also, sometimes opposites will attract, such as the Pineal or Thymus being drawn to the Gonadal or Adrenal.

Returning, specifically, to type considerations as they involve family members, often the foods that can appropriately be eaten by one member will be similar to those acceptable for all members. As an example, let's say that in a particular family of five, all members can handle protein, grains, and vegetables for dinner—while two members can also have fruit. In this case, everyone could participate in the main meal, and the two who could handle fruit would have an additional option.

But what happens when the incompatible foods represent the main part of the meal—say, protein or grains? Balanced and Blood types, for example, do best when carbohydrates are the main emphasis for dinner, so pasta or rice with vegetables would be ideal. Those types who do well with more protein can easily add a protein entrée. A Pituitary woman, married to a Stomach man who needs substantial protein for dinner, can prepare a chicken dinner for the family, eat a light dinner herself (focusing, say, on vegetables and grains), and save her chicken for the next morning. This way, without having to cook two separate meals, she could get her large protein meal for breakfast, and still make it to work on time.

Assuming, however, that you're willing to change any former beliefs about family uniformity, you'll be ready to take the next step. To determine which meals are compatible for family members, check the food groups (protein, grains, vegetables, fruit, nuts, seeds, and dairy) that are the same, then compare the rarely foods for each type and eliminate them. Then you'll be able to plan your joint meals with this information in mind, adding additional entrees as needed for each family member.

Children and Diet

As a parent, you've probably experienced the frustration of having your child refuse to eat something, and not understand what was behind the refusal. Since children are in tune with their bodies (as we ourselves were before we programmed ourselves to ignore them), we need to respect their preferences yet at the same time not allow the child to control us through food. By knowing your child's body type, you know which is which.

Children are very sensitive to foods, and therefore greatly affected by what they eat. Many children will react to sugar, for example, which causes hyperactivity.

When glands, such as the adrenals, are stressed, the first response is hyperactivity, once depleted, they become exhausted. A child's system simply doesn't have the reserves of an adult, so selecting the appropriate foods for each meal becomes an important consideration. If you have a child whose body can't handle fruit in the morning, giving him orange juice will induce a sugar reaction that can look like hyperactivity and result in behavior problems. Or, if you have a child who requires protein for breakfast, not getting it can make him irritable, uncooperative, or hyperactive. There's also the question of what to give a child for a mid-morning snack. For some, fruit or fruit juice is ideal, for others, such a snack will trigger a sugar reaction. Some children are better off with carrot sticks, nuts or seeds; for others, an apple, or a combination of an apple with almond butter is perfect.

When it comes to overall health, what you eat as a child can make the difference between being a healthy adult and someone who suffers from chronic illness. If children are provided with a sound diet that supports their growing bodies, they can handle the dietary abuses of their teen years without succumbing to illnesses. These are the ones who grow up to be healthy adults less prone to illnesses and the effects of aging. Many of the chronically ill adults I work with suffered as children from earaches, headaches, colds, and flu, often having poor dietary choices available to them.

Microwave Cooking

The convenience of microwave cooking has overshadowed a number of studies that show it not to be the benign heating method it's assumed to be.

Microwave cooking is now known to alter the molecular structure of food, producing unhealthful effects. Studies done with breast milk, for example, show that warming it by microwaving causes a breakdown of proteins and antibodies, eliminating the natural infection fighting properties of the milk and destroying its ability to provide the passive immunity it would normally give an infant. This doesn't occur when conventional heating methods are used.

Other studies have shown that eating microwaved foods causes changes in blood chemistry similar to those present in the early stages of cancer. There's an increased tendency toward anemia, elevated cholesterol, and an immune response—as though the microwaved food is an infectious agent.

In addition to altering food molecules so they become difficult to digest or assimilate even under the best of conditions, microwaving destroys the enzymes that would aid in the digestive process. Although any form of cooking will destroy some enzymes, just two seconds of microwave energy destroys all the enzymes in a food.

Microwaved food causes the molecules to move so rapidly that they split in such a way that the body is unable to recognize them as food. The immune system responds to unrecognizable molecules in the same manner as bacteria and viruses, causing the immune system to work overtime. An overactive immune system results in allergies and autoimmune disease.

When food can't be digested fully, it becomes a toxic substance that must be eliminated, and the result is increased stress on the immune system. I often find that people experience a greater incidence of colds and symptoms of a weakened immune system when using a microwave oven.

Weight gain is also common. If the body doesn't have enough energy reserves to eliminate the toxins generated by eating microwaved food, it may gain weight as it stores those toxins in fat cells or suspends them in extracellular fluid. But not all body types react to toxicity in the same way. Some experience weight loss, especially if they normally have a hard time keeping weight on.

Individuals with very strong systems may not be aware of any adverse effects from eating microwaved food, as they are strong enough to absorb the energy drain without any obvious symptoms. However, the immune system is still under stress and will weaken over time. So it's best to avoid using a microwave for any food preparation, even defrosting foods or heating water. Avoiding microwaved food is vitally important for those who have weight problems or trouble with their digestive or immune systems.

Alternative Cooking Methods

I'm always amazed when I tell patients to give up microwave cooking at how many of them will ask me, *"If I don't use the microwave, how can I heat my food?"*

Go back to cooking the way you did before microwaving food became popular. *Steaming* is excellent, and if you don't want the extra moisture, use a *double boiler*. If you're heating food that contains a lot of juices, put it in a dish inside the steamer; this way the juices will stay in the dish.

When you're at work where you don't have a stove, use a portable *hot plate* or *fifth burner*. You can even bring your food in a corning ware dish so you don't have to wash an extra pan.

Toaster ovens are excellent for certain foods, as are *convection ovens*, especially if you want to reduce cooking time.

Leftovers can be heated in a ***skillet***, a ***frying pan***, a ***wok***, or by ***steaming***. When you cook, package the leftovers into individual serving sizes. This is a good way to get away from rut eating, because now when you're hungry you don't have to go to all the work of preparing a healthy meal. Simply take your food out of the freezer and put it in the steamer. This is usually what I do in the mornings for breakfast: I'll put something in the steamer, go take my shower, come back and it's ready.

Exercise Tips

Too busy to exercise? Here are some simple ways to incorporate exercise and body awareness into your daily activities.

Walking. To maintain proper body alignment and get the most out of your steps, focus on using the arch of your foot when you walk. Contact the ground initially with your heel, then roll on to the ball of your foot using the arch of your foot to lift your body. Simply focusing on the arches of your feet as you walk lifts your chest, aligns your spine, and puts a spring into your step.

Sitting. Does your seat get tired from sitting for long periods of time? Do you find yourself crossing your legs or sitting with one foot underneath you? This is your body's way of telling you it needs more space around your tailbone. The bones of your head actually move slightly every time you breathe, acting as a pump to move the cerebral spinal fluid (the fluid that coats the brain and spinal cord) down the spine. The sacrum and tailbone act as a pump to move the fluid back up again to the brain. When the sacrum is unable to move properly, the brain loses alertness and mental clarity. The answer is to sit so your spine can move by using a soft seat or sitting on a large exercise ball.

Using a ***fitness ball*** as a chair not only allows your sacrum to move, it improves posture, reduces wrist problems and strengthens pelvic muscles. The biggest cause of low back pain is lack of flexibility in the lumbar spine and abdominal muscle weakness. Simply sitting on the ball strengthens your pelvic and lower abdominal muscles as well as increases alertness and mental clarity. For additional information on the fitness ball, see *Resources*.

Healthy Food List

Healthy vs. Sensitive Food Lists	This is the *Healthy Food List*. For foods in the *Healthy Food List* that you don't like, don't digest well, or feel sluggish or bloated instead of energized after eating, move them down to a less frequent category. When you feel healthier, you may be able to eat them more often again.

Ultra Support or Frequently Foods
(3-7 meals per week—refers to each food rather than entire category)

Dense Protein Turkey; tuna; calamari (squid), clams, crab, lobster, mussels, oysters; eggs

Cheese Colby, Cheddar, Jack, mozzarella, Romano, raw cheese

Nuts and Seeds Cashews (roasted, unsalted), macadamias, macadamia butter, seeds (caraway, pumpkin, sunflower), sunflower seed butter

Legumes Adzuki or pinto beans

Grains Popcorn, rice (white or brown basmati, long or short grain brown or white), wheat bran, wheat germ, semolina pasta, breads (French, 7-grain, multi-grain)

Vegetables Asparagus, fresh green beans, broccoli, carrots, cabbage (green, napa, red), cauliflower, chard, corn, garlic, leeks, mushrooms, peas, snow pea pods, bell peppers (green, red, yellow), pimentos, potatoes (white rose, russet), pumpkin, sauerkraut

Vegetables Carrot

Fruits Bananas, strawberries, grapes (black, green, red), grapefruits (white, red), oranges, papayas, pineapples, dates, figs (fresh, dried), prunes, raisins, dried fruits

Fruit Juices (Morning) Unfiltered raw apple, pear, grape (purple, red, white), orange

Sweeteners Re-Vita®, stevia

Vegetable Oils Canola, olive, safflower

Beverages Decaf coffee

Basic Support or Moderately Foods
(1-2 meals per week—refers to each food rather than category)

Dense Protein Beef, beef broth, beef liver, buffalo, lamb, ham, pork, bacon, sausage, organ meats (heart, brain), venison, veal; chicken, chicken broth, chicken livers, cornish game hen, duck; anchovy, bass, bonita, catfish, cod, flounder, haddock, halibut, herring, mackerel, mahi-mahi, perch, roughy, salmon, sardines, shark, red snapper, sole, swordfish, trout; abalone, eel, octopus, scallops, shrimp

Healthy Food List

Basic Support or Moderately Foods (cont.)

Dairy
Kefir, plain or flavored yogurt, raw goat milk, milk (whole, 2%, low fat, nonfat, raw), half & half, sweet cream, sour cream, butter, ice cream (Alta Dena®, Breyer's®, Ben & Jerry's®, Dreyer's, Haagen-Dazs®, Swensen's®, Baskin Robbins 31™)

Cheese
American, blue, brie, Camembert, cottage, cream, Edam, feta, raw goat, Gouda, kefir, Limburger, Muenster, Parmesan, ricotta, Swiss, pasteurized cheese

Nuts and Seeds
Almonds, almond butter, Brazils, cashew butter, water chestnuts, coconuts, filberts, hazelnuts, peanuts, peanut butter, pecans, pine nuts, pistachios, walnuts (black, English), sesame seeds, sesame seed butter

Legumes
Beans (black, garbanzo, kidney, navy, great northern, lima [butter], red, soy), lentils, black-eyed peas, split peas, soy milk, tofu, hummus, miso

Grains
Amaranth, barley, buckwheat, corn, corn bread, corn tortillas, hominy grits, millet, oats, quinoa, rice (Japanese, wild, polished), rice bran, rice cakes, triticale, wheat, refined wheat flour, flour tortillas, breads (Italian, garlic, sourdough, white, corn, oat, whole wheat, sprouted grain), croissants, English muffins, crackers (oat, saltines, whole wheat), pasta (whole wheat, corn), couscous, udon noodles, Chinese rice noodles, cream of rice, cream of wheat

Vegetables
Artichokes, arugula, avocados, bamboo shoots, yellow wax beans, lima beans, beets, bok choy, broccoflower, brussels sprouts, celery, cilantro, cole slaw, cucumber, eggplant, greens (beet, collard, mustard, turnip), hominy, jicama, kale, kohlrabi, lettuce (Boston, endive, iceberg, red leaf, romaine), okra, olives (green, ripe), onions (chives, green, brown, red, white, yellow, vidalia), parsley, parsnips, chili peppers, potatoes (red, yukon gold), radish, daikon radish, rutabaga, sauerkraut, seaweed (arame, dulse, kelp, nori, wakame), shallots, spinach, sprouts (alfalfa, mung bean, clover, radish, sunflower), squash (acorn, banana, butternut, spaghetti, yellow [summer], zucchini), sweet potatoes, tomatoes, turnips, watercress, yams

Vegetable Juices
Celery, carrot/celery, parsley, spinach, tomato, V-8®

Fruits
Apples (Golden or Red Delicious, Granny Smith, Jonathan, McIntosh, Pippin, Rome Beauty), apricots, blackberries, blueberries, boysenberries, cranberries, gooseberries, raspberries, cherries, guavas, kiwi, kumquats, lemons, limes, loquats, mangos, melons (casaba, crenshaw, watermelon, honeydew), nectarines, peaches, pears, persimmons, plums (black, purple, red), pomegranates, rhubarb, tangelos, tangerines

Fruit Juices
(Morning) Apple cider, apricot, apple/apricot, black cherry, red cherry, cranapple, cranberry, grapefruit, guava, lemon, papaya, pineapple, pineapple/coconut, prune, tangerine

Healthy Food List

Basic Support or Moderately Foods (cont.)

Vegetable Oils All-blend, almond, avocado, coconut, corn, flaxseed, peanut, sesame, soy, sunflower

Sweeteners Honey, molasses, sorghum, brown sugar, date sugar, raw sugar, refined cane sugar, maple syrup, brown rice syrup, barley malt syrup, corn syrup, fructose, succonant

Condiments Catsup, mustard, horseradish, soy sauce, barbecue sauce, pesto sauce, salsa, tahini, salt, sea salt, Vege-Sal®, vinegar

Salad Dressings Blue cheese, French, ranch, creamy Italian, creamy avocado, thousand island, vinegar and oil, lemon juice and oil

Desserts Custards, tapioca, puddings, pies, cakes, milk chocolate, desserts containing milk chocolate, raspberry sherbet, orange sherbet

Chips Bean, corn (blue, white, yellow), potato

Beverages Coffee; herbal tea, black tea, green tea, Japanese tea, Chinese oolong tea; mineral water, sparkling water; wine (red, white), sake, liqueurs, champagne, beer, barley malt liquor, gin, Scotch, vodka, whiskey; root beer, diet sodas, regular sodas

Stressful or Rarely Foods
(No more than once a month)

Dairy Buttermilk, pasteurized goat milk, most ice creams, frozen yogurt

Cheese Pasteurized goat cheese

Nuts Raw cashews

Grains Rye, rye bread, rye crackers, cream of rye, bagels

Vegetables Butter lettuce

Fruits Cantaloupes

Fruit Juices Filtered, pasteurized apple juice

Healthy Food List

Sweeteners	Saccharin, aspartame, Equal®, NutraSweet®, Sweet'n Low®
Condiments	Mayonnaise, margarine
Desserts	Dark chocolate

Quick Reference Cards Provide a Convenient Format for Your Food Lists

Sensitive Food List

Healthy vs. Sensitive Food Lists	This is the *Sensitive Food List*. It contains all the same foods as the *Healthy Food List*. The difference is that when you are stressed or not digesting well, certain foods should be eaten less often. This list is the extreme – even when fairly stressed you should be able to eat most of these foods more often than stated. See how your body reacts to the foods and adjust accordingly.

Ultra Support or Frequently Foods

(3-7 meals per week—refers to each food rather than entire category)

Nuts and Seeds	Macadamia nuts, pumpkin seeds
Grains	Popcorn
Vegetable	Fresh green beans, carrots
Fruits	Cooked apples, red grapes, oranges, pineapples, papayas, dried bananas
Fruit Juices	Unfiltered raw apple

Basic Support or Moderately Foods

(1-2 meals per week—refers to each food rather than category)

Dense Protein	Beef broth, beef liver, buffalo, veal, venison, lamb, organ meats (heart, brain); turkey, chicken, chicken broth, chicken livers, cornish game hen, duck; anchovy, bass, bonita, catfish, cod, flounder, haddock, halibut, herring, mackerel, mahi-mahi, perch, roughy, salmon, sardines, shark, red snapper, sole, swordfish, trout, tuna; abalone, calamari (squid), clams, crab, eel, lobster, mussels, octopus, oysters, scallops, shrimp; eggs
Dairy	Raw goat milk, half & half, sour cream, sweet cream, kefir, plain or fruit flavored yogurt, butter
Cheese	American, blue, brie, Camembert, Cheddar, Colby, cottage, cream, Edam, feta, raw goat, Gouda, Jack, kefir, Limburger, mozzarella, Muenster, Parmesan, raw cheese, ricotta, Romano, Swiss
Nuts and Seeds	Almond butter, Brazils, cashews (roasted, unsalted), cashew butter, water chestnuts, coconuts, filberts, hazelnuts, macadamia butter, peanuts, peanut butter, pecans, pistachios, pine nuts, walnuts (black, English), seeds (caraway, sesame, sunflower), sesame seed butter, sunflower seed butter
Legumes	Beans (adzuki, black, garbanzo, navy, great northern, kidney, lima [butter], pinto, red), black-eyed peas, split peas, hummus, miso

Sensitive Food List

Basic Support or Moderately Foods (cont.)

Grains
Amaranth, barley, buckwheat, corn, corn bread, corn grits, corn tortillas, hominy grits, millet, oats, quinoa, rice (white or brown basmati, long or short grain brown or white, Japanese, wild), rice bran, rice cakes, refined wheat flour, flour tortillas, breads (French, Italian, garlic, sourdough, 7-grain, multi-grain, oat, corn, rice, sprouted grain), croissants, English muffins, crackers (oat, saltines), couscous, pasta, udon noodles, Chinese rice noodles, cream of rice

Vegetables
Artichokes, asparagus, avocados, bamboo shoots, yellow wax beans, lima beans, beets, bok choy, broccoli, broccoflower, brussels sprouts, cooked cabbage, cauliflower, celery, chard, cilantro, corn, cucumbers, eggplant, garlic, (beet, collard, mustard, turnip), jicama, kale, kohlrabi, leeks, lettuce (Boston, endive, iceberg, red leaf, romaine), mushrooms, okra, olives (green, ripe), onions (chives, green, brown, red, white, yellow, vidalia), parsley, parsnips, peas, snow pea pods, bell peppers (green, red, yellow), chili peppers, pimentos, potatoes (red, russet, white rose), pumpkin, radishes, daikon radishes, rutabaga, seaweed (arame, dulse, kelp, nori, wakame), shallots, spinach, sprouts (alfalfa, clover, mung bean, radish, sunflower), squash (acorn, banana, butternut, spaghetti, yellow [summer], zucchini), sweet potatoes, tomatoes, turnips, yams

Vegetable Juices
Celery, carrot, carrot/celery, parsley, spinach, tomato, V-8®

Fruits
Apples (Golden or Red Delicious, Granny Smith, Jonathan, McIntosh, Pippin, Rome Beauty), apricots, blackberries, blueberries, boysenberries, cranberries, gooseberries, raspberries, strawberries, cherries, green or purple grapes, kiwi, kumquats, limes, loquats, mangos, melons (casaba, crenshaw, honeydew, watermelon), nectarines, pears, persimmons, pomegranates, rhubarb, tangelos, dates, figs, prunes, raisins

Fruit Juices
(Morning) Apple cider, apricot, apple/apricot, red cherry, black cherry, cranapple, cranberry, grape (purple, red, white), guava, orange, papaya, pear, pineapple, pineapple/coconut, prune, tangerine

Vegetable Oils
All-blend, avocado, coconut

Sweeteners
Brown rice syrup, barley malt syrup, Re-Vita®, stevia

Condiments
Salsa, tahini, salt, sea salt, Vege-Sal®, vinegar

Salad Dressings
Vinegar and oil, lemon juice and oil

Beverages
Decaf coffee with Re-Vita®; herbal tea, green tea, Japanese tea, Chinese oolong tea; mineral water, sparkling water

Sensitive Food List

Stressful or Rarely Foods
(No more than once a month)

Dense Protein Beef, ham, pork, bacon, sausage

Dairy Milk (whole, 2%, low fat, nonfat), buttermilk, pasteurized goat milk, most ice creams, frozen yogurt

Cheese Pasteurized goat cheese

Nuts Almonds, raw cashews

Legumes Soy beans, lentils, soy milk, tofu

Grains Polished rice, rye, triticale, whole wheat, wheat bran, wheat germ, breads (rye, white, whole wheat), bagels, crackers (rye, whole wheat), cream of rye, cream of wheat

Vegetables Arugula, raw cabbage, butter lettuce, yukon gold potatoes, sauerkraut, watercress

Fruits Bananas, cantaloupes, grapefruit, lemons, peaches, plums (black, purple, red)

Fruit Juices Filtered pasteurized apple, grapefruit, lemon

Vegetable Oils Almond, canola, corn, flaxseed, olive, peanut, safflower, sesame, soy, sunflower

Salad Dressings Blue cheese, French, ranch, creamy Italian, creamy avocado, thousand island

Sweeteners Honey, molasses, sorghum, raw sugar, refined cane sugar, brown sugar, date sugar, corn syrup, maple syrup, fructose, succonant, saccharin, aspartame, Equal®, Nutra Sweet®, Sweet'n Low®

Condiments Catsup, margarine, mayonnaise, soy sauce, sour pickles, mustard, horseradish, barbecue sauce, pesto sauce

Desserts Custards, tapioca, puddings, pies, cakes, milk chocolate, desserts containing milk chocolate, dark chocolate, raspberry sherbet, orange sherbet

Chips Bean, corn (blue, white, yellow), potato

Beverages Regular coffee; black tea; wine (red, white), sake, liqueurs, beer, barley malt liquor, champagne, gin, Scotch, vodka, whiskey; Pepsi®, root beer, diet sodas, regular sodas

General Dietary Guidelines

THE FOODS LISTED in the various categories are listed for natural, whole-healthy foods. Unfortunately, many foods in the United States have undergone changes that the human body is unable to recognize and process.

- The hybridized process increases **gluten** which stresses the digestive system.

- **Corn** has been genetically modified to kill insects that eat it by destroying the digestive system of the insect and thus, the insect.

Unfortunately, this process also damages the digestive system of animals and humans who eat them. If your digestive system is extremely strong and only a limited amounts of genetically modified products are eaten, you probably will not be aware of their effects. If your system is sensitive, you will want to avoid them.

What are Genetically Modified Organisms - GMOs?

GMOs are living organisms whose genetic material has been artificially manipulated in a laboratory through genetic engineering. This relatively new science creates unstable combinations of plant, animal, bacteria, and viral genes that do not occur in nature or through traditional cross-breeding methods.

What happened to wheat?

In the 1970's wheat underwent hybridization, and in the 1980's genetic modifications reduced its size which increased its yield and that was great for farmers. The changes made it possible for wheat to be used in other ways such as making pastries light, softer and easy to mold into different shapes. Producers realized that the new wheat strain was a potent appetite stimulant. That made it a big seller, and it took over the market place.

Soy is difficult to breakdown for most body types and is almost all GMO. It contains casein which is also found in dairy and difficult for many people to digest.

Dairy is pasteurized and also contains casein. If you are fortunate enough to have a good raw source, evaluate according to your body. Dairy, primarily milk and cheese, are often produced from cattle that have been fed GMO corn, so check your sources. Imported, aged cheeses, sheep or goat cheeses can be good choices. Butter and ghee are excellent fat sources that most people digest well. Kefir is a good probiotic source that can be used to re-establish the intestinal flora after the ingestion of antibiotics. It is possible to experience the effects of antibiotics if you eat commercially raised chicken or meat, like you would typically get when you eat out. Drinking 8 ounces of kefir over the course of 1 to 4 days, will re-establish the food source for the Candida Albicans to maintain a harmonious gut environment. Frequency varies, depending on your system and level of exposure.

General Dietary Guidelines

Sugar: Your intestines are covered with thousands of species of bacteria. The good bugs, or probiotics, work with your body to maintain good digestion. One of the ways the balance of good bugs and bad bugs can get thrown off is by eating too much sugar. When the gut's delicate ecosystem is thrown off, the bad bugs take over and this can result in many chronic illnesses and symptoms. Too much sugar in the diet may lead to diabetes, and is also responsible for a wide-range of health problems. These may include allergies, chronic inflammation, joint problems, digestive symptoms, mood and brain disorders, plus the growth of yeast. Too much yeast in the gut may cause chronic fatigue, loss of energy, general malaise, inability to concentrate, irritability, bloating and gas, frequent bladder infections, and other problems.

Sugar ideally should be limited to 6 tsp or 15 grams per day. This includes natural sugar that is found in fruit. One of the ways we inadvertently get a lot of sugar in our diets is in fruit juice, including smoothies. Dried fruit contains concentrated sugar, and even though it is good sugar, it is easy to mindlessly over-eat, so be aware.

How do I know if I could benefit from eliminating these foods from my diet?

If you suffer from inflammation and chronic pain, migraine headaches, digestive trouble including IBS, bloating, diarrhea or chronic constipation, thyroid issues, Autism, ADD or ADHD or allergies (there are 245 diseases currently associated with food allergies), you may want to start by eliminating the foods that produce the greatest amount of irritation for the greatest number of people. These foods are:

- *Sugar* — particularly refined, white sugar cane.

- *Gluten* — highest source is wheat. If you are extremely sensitive, you may want to start by eliminating all grains. White Basmati rice is the easiest grain to digest and a good place to start when you are reintroducing grains to your diet.

- *Corn* — Blue corn is often a good alternative as is organic popcorn

- *Soy* — almost all soy is now GMO, is hard to digest and contains casein.

- *Dairy* — except for butter - contains casein.

General Dietary Guidelines

If I eliminate all these foods, what am I going to eat?

Primarily **protein** and **vegetables,** along with **good fats**. However, even here you need to be aware. Common vegetables and fruit that are now GMO are zucchini, squash, alfalfa, sugarbeets and papaya.

While salmon is an excellent source of Omega 3 fats, you need to be aware that Atlantic salmon is not wild-caught, but farm-raised.

Fresh young **coconut water** is the closest food to mother's milk. It contains fat, protein, magnesium and acts as a digestive aid. Beware of boxed, canned or processed coconut water; there is a big difference between these and raw fresh young coconut in taste, quality and absorption. Many stores will open the young coconuts for you. Many tools are available online which make opening coconuts yourself easy. To store, pour the coconut water into a glass container with a lid, and add the soft coconut meat. If the meat is soft, you can scrape it out with a spoon. Coconut stores well in the refrigerator for 2 - 4 days or longer. Polarizing your refrigerator can extend the freshness up to 7 or 8 days.

Re-Vita® is spirulina that has been fed minerals, and contains all 22 amino acids. It was developed as an answer for world hunger to be added to milk, and in this combination, reverses symptoms of malnutrition in a few days. I like to add 1 - 2 packets of the Lemon/Lime flavor to the juice of a lemon or two limes into a quart jar and fill it with water. This is great during or after a workout, to sustain your energy throughout the day, a snack, or as a cleanse. During a cleanse, the Re-Vita lemonade can be drunk exclusively throughout the day, or used as a supplement. Re-Vita is sweet and is listed in the Food List under Sweeteners. Add it to oatmeal "cookies", mix it with almond or sunflower seed butter, or make a drink with the berry flavor, cranberry concentrate and water. Put it in your oatmeal along with nuts and butter; add it to butternut squash with cinnamon; or just put it in a spoon and swallow it when you are looking for something sweet to help you digest your meal.

Dietary Guidelines Summary

Focus
- Have a late breakfast with fruit followed by protein
- Avoid fruit for lunch and dinner
- Lunch on raw vegetables, salads, nuts, and seeds (raw vegetables best assimilated at lunch)
- Make dinner a cooked meal with steamed vegetables
- Emphasize vegetables, fruit, cheese, nuts, and soups

Dietary Emphasis
- Fats: 25 to 30 percent of total calories
- Best fat sources: avocados, seeds (pumpkin, sunflower, and sesame), tahini, and nuts (almonds, pecans, Brazils, coconut, macadamias, pistachios, and dry-roasted cashews)
- Total protein: 20 to 35 percent of calories from protein
- Dense protein: 0 to 25 percent of calories from dense protein
- Caloric intake: 1,500 to 1,800 calories a day for women and 1,700 to 2,000 calorie a day for men. If you are engaging in intense exercise (competition type) or heavy labor, increase calories
- Drink a minimum of 64 ounces of water a day. Drink water before and after meals, not with meals
- To detoxify system, drink herbal tea or hot water with lemon upon rising. Wait 2 to 3 hours before eating breakfast
- Occasional desserts are best as an evening snack
- Cooked vegetables are best for dinner
- Broccoli, zucchini, and yellow squash should always be eaten raw
- Eat more raw vegetables than cooked
- Rotate foods

Weight Loss
- Protein: 15 to 25 percent of daily calories
- Protein and fruit for breakfast at least 2 times a week
- Limit dairy, cheese, frozen yogurt, fried foods, alcohol, caffeine, diet sodas, and breads with yeast
- Limit snack to evening
- May skip lunch and have light snack at midafternoon or wen hungry
- Adhere to time schedule for meals: *breakfast 9–10am, lunch 1–2pm, dinner 6:30–9pm*

Weight Gain
- *Fat:* 35 percent of daily calories. Emphasize dairy, avocados, nuts, and seeds
- *Dense protein:* 15 to 25 percent of daily calories
- Consume protein and fruit for breakfast
- Increase quantity of food and include snacks
- Exercise is essential to build muscle weight

Dietary Guidelines Summary

Vegetarian Diet

Recommended when healthy, although diet may consist of up to 20 percent dense protein

Amino Acids

Best sources of the amino acids threonine, isoleucine and cystine are turkey, tuna, and pumpkin seeds

Fats

Fats: 25 to 30 percent of total calories. *Best fat sources:* avocados, coconuts, seeds (pumpkin, sunflower, and sesame), tahini, and nuts (almonds, pecans, Bazils, macadamias, pistachios, and dry-roasted cashews)

Menu Key

These menus have been tested for ease of digestion and optimal nutritional support. The food combination consist of basic foods, allowing for complementary spices to be used to suit your taste. If desired, additional dishes may be included to enhance a meal. You will notice that some menu items are designated "A", "L", "S" & "G" *(see below)*. Some menu items are "L" or "G" while others have any one or a combination of designations.

"A" is for *adrenal rebuilding*. When the adrenal glands have become exhausted, the body needs additional support particularly at breakfast and lunch. The main adrenal rebuilding foods are protein and vegetables with limited fruit eaten at the specified time of day for your body type.

"L" is specifically for *weight loss*.

"S" is for *sensitive* and means this combination is very easy to digest and can be selected when you don't want to devote a lot of energy to digesting your meal, such as when you are fighting a cold or are under a lot of stress.

"G" is for *weight gain* or when you want to build extra muscle mass. Many times the menu is the same for both weight loss and weight gain because both much and too little weight are signs of the body being out of balance. The solution is the same—a diet that provides the nutrients you need to truly support your body.

When you are at your ideal weight you may choose from all of the menus. All menus may be used by healthy persons.

() around foods means these foods are *optional*.

Menus

A = *adrenal rebuilding*   **L** = *weight loss*
S = *sensitive*   **G** = *weight gain*   **( )** = *optional*
(See previous page for more info on menu key)

BREAKFAST

9-10 a.m. Light, with protein, dairy, and/or fruit.

SENSITIVE: *Light-to-moderate, with fruit, protein, dairy, and/or grain..*

S G	Eggs and grape juice
S G	Eggs and fruit (toast)
S G	Scrambled eggs w/cheese, or cheese omelette
L	Basted eggs and grapefruit
L	Hard-boiled egg and fruit juice
	Bacon or ham, and pineapple or pineapple juice
A L G	Chicken or cornish hen, w/grapes or white grape juice
L G	Chicken w/pineapple chunks or pineapple juice
A L G	Turkey w/apples, applesauce, or unfiltered apple juice
A L G	Duck and cherries
L	Tuna w/lemon juice
A L G	Lobster and grapes, apples, cherries, or blackberries
A L G	Mussels and apples
A L G	Oysters and grapes
S G	Cottage cheese and pineapple, or green apples
G	Plain yogurt and apple or banana
S G	Nonfat raspberry yogurt
S G	Yogurt or kefir and berry Re-Vita®
S	Oatmeal w/raisins and butter
S	Granola or muesli w/kefir
S	Rice w/butter
S	Basmati rice and mango, or papaya (plain yogurt)
S	Couscous w/blackberries, blueberries, raspberries, or Re-Vita®
S	Raisin bread toast and butter
S	5-grain pancakes w/apple sauce
S	Pancakes w/blueberries or strawberries and Re-Vita®
S	Waffles and strawberries or blueberries (Re-Vita®)
S	Baked apple w/cinnamon
S	Grape juice

MID-MORNING SNACK

(Optional) Grain, vegetables, fruit, dairy, nuts, seeds, protein, and/or legumes.

L	Carrot and beet juice
G	Celery w/almond butter
S	Popcorn, unsalted (parmesan cheese)
G	Coconut
S G	Peanuts, walnuts, pistachios, sunflower seeds
G	Raw or roasted sunflower or pumpkin seeds, unsalted
S	Pumpkin seeds and raisins
S	Oat crackers and cheese .
	Granola bar
	Pineapple/coconut juice

LUNCH

1-2 p.m. Moderate, with grain, raw vegetables, legumes, dairy, nuts, and/or seeds.

SENSITIVE: *Moderate, w/ protein, dairy, and/or vegetables.*

G	Corn tortilla, refried beans, and kefir or feta cheese
G	Corn tortilla and mozzarella cheese
G	Flour tortilla, cheese, and avocado
L	Pasta or couscous w/butter
L	Pasta and raw broccoli (Italian dressing)
L	Pasta w/pesto and raw carrots
G	Chicken taquito w/guacamole and cheese
	Spinach lasagna and salad: romaine lettuce, tomato, cucumber, red bell pepper w/creamy Italian dressing

Menus

LUNCH (con't)

A S		Chicken, potatoes, and raw broccoli or spinach
A L S		Chicken, raw broccoli, and corn
A S		Orange roughy and raw broccoli or green beans
	S G	Sole fillet, scalloped potatoes, and raw spinach
	S	Tuna and salad w/oil and vinegar or salad dressing
	S	Tuna and sunflower seed sprouts
A L S		Salmon, cauliflower, and raw broccoli or salad
A L S		Salmon and salad: cucumber, spinach, and green peas
A S G		Salmon, red leaf lettuce, cucumber, carrots, and tomatoes w/creamy Italian dressing
A S		Lamb chops, peas, and mushrooms
	S	Steak, mushrooms, onions, and raw carrots
	G	English muffin w/avocado or peanut butter and honey
	G	Peanut butter and Re-Vita® sandwich
	G	Oatmeal muffin w/butter and swiss cheese
	G	Sourdough bread, Jack cheese, and jicama w/Creamy Italian dressing
		Celery w/peanut butter and carrots
	G	Baked potato topped w/mozzarella cheese (sprouts)
		Baked potato w/melted cheese and raw broccoli
	G	Vegetable pasta and cream sauce
L		Bean burrito w/avocado or salad and low fat dressing
L		Bean burrito and salad: red leaf or romaine lettuce, tomato, onion, and mushrooms
	G	Pizza, cheese, (black olives), and raw carrots
	G	Vegetarian pizza w/cheese (salad)
	S	Corn tortilla and Jarlsburg cheese
L		Spinach salad
	G	Spinach salad w/sunflower or pumpkin seeds

L S	Spinach leaves, cucumber, sesame oil, and sprouts
L	3-bean salad and red leaf lettuce salad
S	Salad: jicama, carrots, red bell peppers, green onions, and spinach w/blue cheese dressing
S	Chef salad: 3 cheeses, turkey, romaine lettuce, alfalfa sprouts, and cherry tomatoes
L	Salad: romaine lettuce, alfalfa sprouts, cherry tomatoes, seeds, and ranch dressing
	Cobb salad
S	Chicken w/rice and noodle soup
L S	Carrot and beet juice
S	Plain kefir

MID-AFTERNOON SNACK

(Optional) 4 p.m. Dairy, nuts, seeds, grain, and/or vegetables.

S	String cheese
S	Rice cakes or rice crackers w/mozzarella cheese
G	Muffin
G	Bread with tahini butter
G	Nuts and/or seeds
G	Protein bar
G	Cookies

DINNER

6:30-9 p.m. Moderate, with protein, dairy, legumes, cooked or steamed vegetables, and/or grain. Raw vegetables, as in salads, may be consumed with meat and pasta.

Sensitive: *7-9 p.m. Moderate, with grain, dairy, legumes, and/or vegetables.*

A L		Turkey, white rose potatoes, and green beans
L	G	Turkey, mashed potatoes, and mixed vegetables
		Turkey, pickle, lettuce, tomato, and mustard on whole wheat bread
		Curry chicken w/rice and pasta – egg noodles or semolina

Menus

DINNER *(con't)*

	Dish
	Chicken, pasta, and garlic sauce
L	Chicken, spinach, and red potatoes
A L G	Cashew chicken, water chestnuts, snow pea pods, and rice
A L	Chicken, rice, and green beans or asparagus or peas
A L G	Chicken, corn and broccoli or cole slaw
A L G	Chicken, pasta, and broccoli
L G	Barbecued chicken and Chinese vegetables
G	Chicken taquito w/guacamole and cheese
G	Chicken, lettuce, cheese, and sauce on tortilla
	Chicken toastada
A L	Chicken, pinto beans, and rice (butternut squash)
L G	Orange chicken, rice, and chow mein
	Chow mein, fried rice, hot and sour soup, and steamed vegetables
G	Sausage, pasta (cooked celery, green onions, and/or red and green peppers)
G	Steak and pasta (salad)
G	Barbecued steak, mushrooms, onions, and carrots
G	Corned beef and sauerkraut
G	Carne asada burrito w/beef and guacamole (salad)
L G	Lamb chops, peas, and mushrooms
G	Swordfish, scalloped potatoes, and leeks
A L	Cod, rice pilaf, and asparagus
A L G	Rainbow trout, pasta, and raw broccoli
A L	Halibut and asparagus
G	Halibut, pasta, and salad
A L	Salmon, basmati rice, and asparagus
G	Salmon and flour tortilla (salad or vegetable)
L	Barbecued salmon, broccoli or salad, and cauliflower
L G	Red snapper, pasta, and asparagus
	Shrimp, tomato garlic pasta, and green beans
	Shrimp, green beans, and tomato garlic pasta
S	Pasta or couscous w/butter
S G	Pasta w/pesto
G	Pasta w/clam sauce
G	Pasta, Parmesan cheese, and broccoli
L G	Pasta, olive oil, garlic, and spices (zucchini, cauliflower and broccoli, or cauliflower and green beans, or asparagus and carrots)
L	Pasta w/tomato marinara, mushrooms, and onions
S G	Spaghetti (Parmesan cheese) and meat balls
S	Spinach lasagna and salad: lettuce, tomato, cucumber, red bell pepper w/creamy Italian dressing
G	Tofu, macaroni, and broccoli
G	Tofu lasagna
S	Corn tortilla w/avocado
G	Tamales (soy cheese), (rice)
L S	Brown rice and steamed vegetables
S	Rice and beans
S	Refried beans and corn tortilla
	Adzuki beans and rice (curry)
L	Lentils, onions, peppers (rice, beans, or cauliflower)
L	Pizza and hot spiced carrots
L G	Hawaiian pizza w/ham and pineapple
G	Pizza, cheese (pepperoni), (black olives), and carrots (antipasta vegetable salad)
G	Pizza w/tomato sauce, mozzarella cheese, and salad
G	Vegetarian pizza w/cheese
L S	Stir-fry: mushrooms, onions, carrots, celery, red peppers, and pasta
L S	Stir-fry: Chinese vegetables and rice
S	Baked pumpkin w/butter and cinnamon
S	Spaghetti squash and green peas
S	Carrots and cooked cabbage
S	Potatoes and sour cream
S G	Yams, peas, and butter

Menus

DINNER *(con't)*

G	Chili and cornbread
S	Oatmeal
S	Soup: cabbage, endive, and leek (onion)
L S	Soup: red potatoes, cauliflower, and beets
L S	Split pea soup
L S	Bean soup
L	Beef broth or chicken broth w/vegetables
L	Chicken noodle soup
	Chicken vegetable soup

EVENING SNACK

(Optional) 10 p.m.-1 a.m. Protein, dairy, vegetables, grain, nuts, seeds, sweets.

Sensitive: *9-11 p.m. Fruit, grain, sweets.*

	Rice cake and nut butter
G	Peanuts, walnuts, pistachios, roasted cashews, or sunflower seeds
L	Popcorn (olive oil)
S G	Milk chocolate
G	Cake
S G	Pumpkin pie
G	Apple pie 1 hour after dinner
S	Fruits: nectarine, pear, grapes, apple, or figs
G	Dates or figs
S	Sorbet w/strawberries, blueberries, or raspberries
S	Toasted sourdough bread w/butter (before bed)

One Week Sample Menu

DAY 1 **BREAKFAST**
Grapes or white grape juice, then chicken breast

LUNCH
Pasta w/raw broccoli and Italian dressing

SNACK
Raw carrots and sunflower seeds

DINNER
Steak, potatoes, and salad of spinach, potatoes, and green onions w/balsamic vinegar and olive oil

DAY 2 **BREAKFAST**
Orange, then mushroom and egg omelette

LUNCH
Tomato, avocado, and onion w/balsamic vinegar and oil over Boston lettuce and couscous

DINNER
Split pea soup and French bread w/butter

DAY 3 **BREAKFAST**
Bananas, then cottage cheese

LUNCH
Falafel, rice, and a salad of green leaf lettuce, feta cheese, onions, and Greek salad and bell pepper with olive oil and vinegar dressing

SNACK
Kefir

DINNER
Salmon, basmati rice, and asparagus

DAY 4 **BREAKFAST**
Cantaloupe, then a salad of chicken, grapes, walnuts, and celery

LUNCH
Bean burrito and a salad of red leaf or romaine lettuce, tomato, onion, and mushrooms

DINNER
Fillet of tuna and basmati rice w/leeks, snow pea pods, and bell peppers

DAY 5 **BREAKFAST**
Cherries and duck

LUNCH
Celery with peanut butter and carrots

DINNER
Rainbow trout and brussels sprouts

DAY 6 **BREAKFAST**
Grapes, then hard-boiled eggs

LUNCH
Salad of romaine lettuce, alfalfa sprouts, cherry tomatoes, and pumpkin seeds w/ranch dressing

DINNER
Teriyaki chicken rice bowl and vegetables such as broccoli, carrots, celery, snow pea pods, bamboo shoots w/soy sauce

DAY 7 **BREAKFAST**
Orange juice, cheese omelette

LUNCH
Orange roughy and green beans

DINNER
Turkey, White Rose potatoes, and green beans

Alternative Menu Items

BREAKFAST

Grapefruit and eggs

Apples, applesauce, or unfiltered apple juice and turkey
Grapes or apples and lobster

Cherries or blackberries and lobster

Apples and mussels

Grapes and oysters

Pineapple chunks or pineapple juice and chicken

Apple, then ham or pork chops

Pineapple and cottage cheese

LUNCH

Pasta w/pesto sauce and raw carrots

Salmon, cauliflower, and raw broccoli

Salmon and a salad of cucumber, spinach, and green peas

Bean burrito w/avocado

Three-bean salad on red leaf lettuce

Chef's salad of turkey, romaine lettuce, alfalfa sprouts, and cherry tomatoes with ranch dressing

DINNER

Chicken, spinach, and red potatoes

Cashew chicken, water chestnuts, snow pea pods, and rice

Halibut and asparagus

Red snapper, pasta, and asparagus

Rainbow trout, pasta, and asparagus

Rice and beans (cheese enchilada w/avocado, salsa)

Scrambled eggs w/broccoli

Lentils, onions, and peppers (rice, beans, or cauliflower)

Stir-fried mushrooms, onions, carrots, celery, red peppers, and pasta

Bean soup

Chicken noodle soup

SNACKS

Yogurt and pecans

Cottage cheese and pineapple (tomato)

Raisins and nuts (oatmeal)

Macadamia nuts and apricots

Potato, lettuce, and/or avocado

Peanuts and raisins

Almonds and dried cherries

Celery w/peanut butter

Cottage cheese w/pineapple

Sample Cleanse Menu

Ideally cleanse to 3 days, 1 to 4 times per month. Items in parenthesis ( ) are optional.

BREAKFAST

Watermelon whole w/seeds and white part of rine

LUNCH

Raw carrots, bell pepper, jicama, celery with olive oil and vinegar and/or juice of carrot or carrot/celery (parsley/spinach)

DINNER

Steamed broccoli and/or cauliflower, green beans, corn (no butter)

Protein Powders and Supplements

When and how often to use protein powders, bars and food supplements with specific options for different times of day. Supplements are listed with most supportive first. Food items in parentheses () are optional.

ON RISING *(Choose one)*

NingXia Red™

Total Body Greens™

BREAKFAST *(Choose one)*

Whole Body Collagen™

Balance Complete™

Premier Whey Protein™ with almond milk, rice milk or fruit juice
   (blueberries, fruit)

Lean Advantage™

Pure Protein Complete

Premier Nutritional Flakes™

Phytotein™

MID-MORNING SNACK *(Choose one)*

Whole Body Collagen™

NingXia Red™

Re-Vita™ with cranberry concentrate, lemon or lime juice and water

Premier Whey Protein™ with fruit juice
   (blueberries, fruit)

PurePaleo Bone Broth

Lean Advantage™

Premier Nutritional Flakes™

Premier Plant Protein™

LUNCH

Natural food

MID-AFTERNOON SNACK *(Choose one)*

Premier Whey Protein™ with fruit juice
   (blueberries, fruit)

Lean Advantage™

Premier Nutritional Flakes™

Whole Body Collagen™

PurePaleo Bone Broth

Phytotein™

Premier Plant Protein™

Total Body Greens™

NingXia Red™

DINNER *(Choose one)*

Whole Body Collagen™

Balance Complete™

Premier Nutritional Flakes™

EVENING SNACK *(Choose one)*

Whole Body Collagen™

Re-Vita with cranberry concentrate, lemon or lime juice and water

Premier Nutritional Flakes™

Designs for Health Bar™

Protein Powders and Supplements

NUTRITIONAL SUPPORT

(maximum weekly servings per supplement)

Young Living Essential Oils

(See your Young Living representative for these supplements):

Balance Complete™ - 5 times weekly

NingXia Red™ - 7 times weekly

Power Meal™ - once weekly

Pure Protein Complete™ - 3 times weekly

Body Type Store

(Scan the QR code below for these supplements):

Designs for Health Bar™ - 3 times weekly

Lean Advantage™ - 2 times weekly

Phytotein™ - 3 times weekly

Premier Nutritional Flakes™ - 7 times weekly

Premier Plant Protein™ - 2 times weekly

Premier Whey Protein™ - up to twice daily, 4 days per week

PurePaleo Bone Broth™ - 3 times weekly

Re-Vita™ - 7 times weekly

Total Body Greens™ - 4 times weekly

Whole Body Collagen™ - 7 times weekly

Re-Vita with cranberry concentrate, lemon or lime juice and water

Designs for Health Bar™

Pure Protein Complete

Power Meal™

Visit BodyType.com.

Resources

PROTEIN POWDERS

Balance Complete™
by Young Living Essential Oils®

A daily nutrient and cleanse meal replacement containing 11 grams fiber, whey protein and Ningxia wolfberries.

Lean Advantage™
by Premier Research Labs®

Supports weight management, lean body mass and glycemic metabolism. World-class, full-spectrum ingredients include Green Coffee Bean Extract, Raspberry Ketones, and Citrus Aurantium extract – which helps promote fat breakdown.

Phytotein™
by Designs for Health®

Phytotein provides 20 grams of vegan plant-based protein and the amino acid lysine. This organic blend includes high quality non-GMO pea protein supplemented with sunflower, pumpkin seed, sacha inchi, and rice sources. A tasty and easily digestible alternative for those sensitive to dairy, gluten, whey, casein and soy. Available in chocolate and vanilla flavors.

Power Meal Vegan Meal Replacement™
by Young Living Essential Oils®

This nutrient-dense shake provides 20 grams of plant protein for powering through your day. 11 fruits and vegetables are enhanced with a dash of orange essential oil and vanilla. Rich in amino acids with zero added sugar. A balanced meal with fats, carbohydrates, protein and fiber, including 17 vitamins and minerals. Only 170 calories per serving.

Premier Nutritional Flakes™
by Premier Research Labs®

A quality source of vegan protein with a pleasant, cheesy taste. Non-GMO yeast provides bioavailable protein rich in B vitamins and amino acids. Sprinkle on salads, soups and other dishes for a hearty, cheesy taste. Only 40 calories per serving.

Premier Plant Protein™
by Premier Research Labs®

An organic, vegan protein powder including pea, which has been shown to subdue ghrelin, which sends hunger signals to the brain. Naturally free of allergens and ideal for those with food sensitivities. Provides 18 grams of protein. Supplies over 60 trace minerals without any synthetic ingredients.

Premier Whey Protein™
by Premier Research Labs®

Premier whey protein is a highly nutritious protein containing all 17 of the essential and non-essential amino acids. Premier's whey formula is guaranteed pesticide free, is produced using ultrafiltration at a very low temperature to preserve the broad array of protein molecules, including naturally occurring glycomacropeptides (GMPs) and is not toxic to the kidneys. It's great taste makes a wonderful smoothie or shake.

PurePaleo Bone Broth Protein™
by Designs for Health®

Contains a highly concentrated pure beef protein, produced through an exclusive hydrolysis and ultra filtration process. This process begins with beef from animals raised in Sweden, without hormones and free of any GMO grasses, grains, and ensilage. This purified beef protein contains both complete and collagen proteins that are naturally found in beef. Ideal for those who are dairy sensitive and want to build muscle, cartilage and ligaments from a true Paleo protein source. Comes in chocolate and vanilla flavors.

Resources

Pure Protein Complete™
by Young Living Essential Oils®

A whey-based protein drink designed to increase energy, strengthen the immune system, and build lean muscle mass. Flavors: Vanilla Spice and Chocolate.

Whole Body Collagen™
by Designs for Health®

Contains a unique blend of three patented collagen peptides supporting collagen production, bone strength, joint health and skin elasticity. Can be incorporated into shakes, smoothies, and other foods and beverages.

SUPER FOODS

NingXia Red™
by Young Living Essential Oils®

Made from Ningxia wolfberries. Provides dynamic energy and stamina without harmful stimulants. This anti-aging antioxident has the highest levels of ORAC activity. Supports the immune system, vision and liver. Visit **www.ningxiared.com** for information.

Re-Vita®
by Re-Vita®, Inc.

Spirulina that has been fed minerals and contains all 22 of the amino acids. May be used as a supplement or as a meal replacement once or twice a day. It comes in syrup form and is sweet. The average serving is 1 tablespoon.

Total Body Greens™
by World Health Mall™

An easy mixing, great tasting and energizing "phyto-nutrient" powder mix loaded with certified organic whole foods and plant extracts. Comes in original, berry, and chocolate with pure organic cocoa.

NUTRITIONAL BARS

Protein Bar™
by Designs for Health®

Small meal options, pre/post workout and be¬tween meal snacks. Optimal macronutrient blend for sustained energy and hunger control.

- *Bone Broth Chocolate Crunch Bar*
- *Cocommune Supplement Bar*
- *Peanut Butter Joint Power Protein Bar*
- *Yes Whey!! Ultimate Protein Bar*
- *Bold Beauty Collagen Protein Bar*
- *Plant-Powered Magnesium Protein Bar*

Resources

OTHER FOODS

Coconut Oil
By Tropical Traditions®

Coconut oil is one of the best cooking oils to use and is rich in lauric acid which supports the immune system. It is unrefined, organic, no trans fatty acids, and provides energy which can lead to weight loss.

Pink Salt
By Premier Research Labs®

Unrefined, untreated sea salt containing valuable trace elements not found in regular table salt.

VIBRATIONALS

Father Genetics & Mother Genetics

While in utero and during infancy, we pick up emotions, attitudes, and perspectives from our parents and their genetic lines that we collect and adopt as our own. Some of these we would like to keep, while many of these can be hindrances to where we want to be in life. Father Genetics and Mother Genetics bring to your awareness where these patterns come from and allow you to consciously decide if you want to keep them, adapt them, transmute them or simply release them.

PRODUCTS

EMF Neutralizer (for cellphones) – Puts a positive energy field around the phone, neutralizing potentially harmful radiation. May also be used on devices such as computers, portable phones, or digital watches.

Living Water House System – Makes water taste good, helps dry skin and helps hydration of cells. De-scales plumbing and enhances plant growth.

Living Water Pool Patch – Makes skin softer, decreases stinging eyes and fading clothes. Reduces scale build-up, making cleaning easier and makes equipment last longer.

Chakra Harmony DVD – This easy to follow DVD will show you how to balance your life energies and relieve stress. Can be used actively or as a soothing background for relaxing and revitalizing yourself and others. Suitable for all ages, combines visual and sound toning techniques to harmonize your body, mind and spirit.

Chakra Essential Oils Kit – Safety pack with eight Chakra Essential Oils. For added enhancement, combine the Chakra Harmony DVD with the eight recommended Essential Chakra Oils to further your awareness of your healing senses.

EXERCISE

Fitness Ball – The easiest way to exercise. Incorporate exercise into your lifestyle by using a fitness ball as a chair. The weakest point of the body is the pelvis which results in weakness of the lower abdominal muscles and low back pain. Sitting on the ball forces you to use your pelvic and lower abdominal muscles. This improves posture, reduces wrist problems, and stimulates cerebral-spinal fluid movement, resulting in increased alertness and mental clarity.

Core Fitness DVD – Focuses on effectively strengthening the abdominal muscles with the Pilates-based exercises using the Fitness Ball. The 60 minute DVD includes a 40 minute workout on the Fitness Ball, a mini workout that targets your weakest areas, and exercises that can be done at your desk while sitting on the ball.

Resources

RELATED WORKS

Releasing Emotional Patterns with Essential Oils
– by Carolyn L. Mein, D.C., Vision Ware Press. Clear deep-seated, emotional patterns permanently with quick and easy techniques.

Excitotoxins: The Taste That Kills –
– by Dr. Russell Blaylock, neurosurgeon, Health Press (1-800-643-2665).

Defense Against Alzheimer's
– by Dr. H.J. Roberts, diabetic specialist (1-800-814-9800).

For more information on aspartame:

- www.aspartamekills.com
- www.dorway.com

CONTACT INFORMATION

To order, or for additional information, contact your health care professional, nutritionist or local distributor. Or contact us directly.

Phone: (858) 756-3704

Fax: (858) 756-6933

Online: www.bodytype.com

Visit BodyType.com and click SHOP

Body Type Products

Books

Different Bodies, Different Diets™ — Women's Edition & Men's Edition. These two dietary and body typing guides are based on more than 20 years of research. The **25 Body Type System**™ was created to optimize health and vitality. Following the diet designed to support their body has allowed people who have tried diet after diet, with little success, to take off excess weight and keep it off. Actual photos of real-life people provide realistic pictures of what your body would look like if you were overweight, underweight, or at your ideal weight. This book allows readers to determine their body type and to then discover the specific diet most appropriate for them.

Different Bodies, Different Diets™ — Combined Edition. This edition published by HarperCollins contains photos of both men and women. Celebrities are referenced for each body type, along with one week sample menus.

Releasing Emotional Patterns with Essential Oils — A practical guide to the use of specific essential oils for clearing emotional patterns. It contains over 500 common emotions from "fear of abandonment" to "worry". Also included are charts showing the location of body alarm points, as well as reflex points on the hands and feet.

Additional Body Type Publications

Body Type Profiles and Diets - 25 Individual Booklets
Body Type Questionnaire - Men and Women
25 Body Type Photos - Men and Women
Microwaves & Dietary Myths
Advanced Dietary Guide
Body Type Essences
Muscle Testing

DVDs & CDs

Body Type Interviews (DVD) — Contains TV interviews of Dr. Mein on News 13 Los Angeles, New Attitudes, Inside Edition, KUSI News, Channel 10 News, KABC Los Angeles, KTLA Los Angeles and Southland Today. Ideal introduction to the body type system – great for patients and clients.

Core Fitness (DVD) — Focuses on effectively strengthening the abdominal muscles and pelvic floor with Pilates-based exercises using the Fitness-Fun-Ball™. Includes exercises you can do at your desk using the Fitness-Fun-Ball™ as a chair.

Chakra Harmony (DVD) — Harmonize your body, mind and spirit with essential oils and toning.

Body Type Training Seminar (CD) — Contains 6 CD's of live training seminar showing how to determine 25 different body types.

For Seminars, Lectures, Certification or Professionals in your Area

Call **(858) 756-3704** or visit our website at **www.bodytype.com**